Cardiovascular
Physiology

Cardiovascular Physiology

7th edition

David E. Mohrman, PhD
Associate Professor
Department of Physiology and Pharmacology
University of Minnesota Medical School
Duluth, Minnesota

Lois Jane Heller, PhD
Professor
Department of Physiology and Pharmacology
University of Minnesota Medical School
Duluth, Minnesota

 Medical

New York   Chicago   San Francisco   Lisbon   London   Madrid   Mexico City
Milan   New Delhi   San Juan   Seoul   Singapore   Sydney   Toronto

Cardiovascular Physiology, Seventh Edition

2 3 4 5 6 7 8 9 0   DOC/DOC   14 13 12 11 10

ISBN 978-0-07-170120-4
MHID 0-07-170120-6
ISSN 1541-9002

This book was set in Adobe Garamond by Aptara, Inc.
The editors were Michael Weitz and Christie Naglieri.
The production supervisor was Sherri Souffrance.
Project management was provided by Indu Jawwad, Aptara, Inc.
The cover designer was Gazillion Group.
The indexer was Aptara, Inc.
RR Donnelley was printer and binder.

This book is printed on acid-free paper.

McGraw-Hill books are available at special quantity discounts to use as premiums and sales promotions, or for use in corporate training programs. To contact a representative, please e-mail us at bulksales@mcgraw-hill.com.

Contents

Preface

This text is intended to give beginning medical and serious physiology students a strong understanding of the basic operating principles of the intact cardiovascular system. In the course of their careers, these students will undoubtedly encounter a blizzard of new research findings, drug company claims, etc. Our basic rationale is that to be able to evaluate such new information, one must understand where it fits in the overall picture.

In many curricula, the study of cardiovascular physiology is a student's first exposure to a complete organ system. Many students who have become masters at memorizing isolated facts understandably have some difficulty in adjusting their mindset to think and reason about a system as a whole. We have attempted to foster this transition with our text and challenging study questions. In short, our goal is to have students "understand" rather than "know" cardiovascular physiology.

We are also conscious of the fact that cardiovascular physiology is allotted less and less time in most curricula. We have attempted to keep our monograph as short and succinct as possible. Our goal from the first edition onward has been to help students understand how the "bottom-line" principles of cardiovascular operations apply to the various physiological and pathological challenges that occur during everyday life. Thus, our monograph is aimed throughout with its last two chapters in mind. These chapters bring together the individual components to show how the overall system operates under normal and abnormal situations. We judged what facts to include in the beginning chapters on the basis of whether they needed to be referred to in these last two chapters.

In this seventh edition, we have attempted to hone our fundamental approach through more precise language, better organization of some of the material, incorporation of a few new factual updates that clarify our understanding of basic concepts, and inclusion of additional thought-provoking study questions.

As always, we wish to express sincere thanks to our mentors while we were students and to our own students for all the things they have taught us over the years.

David E. Mohrman, PhD
Lois Jane Heller, PhD

Overview of the Cardiovascular System

OBJECTIVES

The student understands the homeostatic role of the cardiovascular system, the basic principles of cardiovascular transport, and the basic structure and function of the components of the system.

▶ *Defines homeostasis.*

▶ *Identifies the major body fluid compartments and states the approximate volume of each.*

▶ *Lists three conditions, provided by the cardiovascular system, that are essential for regulating the composition of interstitial fluid (ie, the internal environment).*

▶ *Diagrams the blood flow pathways between the heart and other major body organs.*

▶ *States the relationship among blood flow, blood pressure, and vascular resistance.*

▶ *Predicts the relative changes in flow through a tube caused by changes in tube length, tube radius, fluid viscosity, and pressure difference.*

▶ *Identifies the chambers and valves of the heart and describes the pathway of blood flow through the heart.*

▶ *Defines cardiac output.*

▶ *Describes the pathway of action potential propagation in the heart.*

▶ *Lists the five factors essential to proper ventricular pumping action.*

▶ *States the relationship between ventricular filling and cardiac output (Starling's law of the heart) and describes its importance in the control of cardiac output.*

▶ *Identifies the distribution of sympathetic and parasympathetic nerves in the heart and lists the basic effects of these nerves on the heart.*

▶ *Lists the major different types of vessels in a vascular bed and describes the morphological differences among them.*

▶ *Describes the basic anatomical features and function of the different vessel types.*

▶ *Identifies the major mechanisms in vascular control and blood flow distribution.*

▶ *Describes the basic composition of the fluid and cellular portions of blood.*

HOMEOSTATIC ROLE OF THE CARDIOVASCULAR SYSTEM

A 19th-century French physiologist, Claude Bernard (1813–1878), first recognized that all higher organisms actively and constantly strive to prevent the external environment from upsetting the conditions necessary for life within the organism.

Thus, the temperature, oxygen concentration, pH, ionic composition, osmolarity, and many other important variables of our *internal environment* are closely controlled. This process of maintaining the "constancy" of our internal environment has come to be known as *homeostasis*. To accomplish this task, an elaborate material transport network, the cardiovascular system, has evolved.

Three compartments of watery fluids, known collectively as the *total body water*, account for approximately 60% of body weight. This water is distributed among the *intracellular, interstitial,* and *plasma* compartments, as indicated in Figure 1–1. Note that about two-thirds of our body water is contained within cells and communicates with the interstitial fluid across the plasma membranes of cells. Of the fluid that is outside cells (ie, extracellular fluid), only a small amount, the *plasma volume*, circulates within the cardiovascular system. Blood is composed of plasma and roughly an equal volume of formed elements (primarily red cells). The

Figure 1–1. Major body fluid compartments with average volumes indicated for a 70-kg human. Total body water is approximately 60% of body weight.

circulating plasma fluid communicates with the interstitial fluid across the walls of small capillary vessels within organs.

The interstitial fluid is the immediate environment of individual cells. (It is the "internal environment" referred to by Bernard.) These cells must draw their nutrients from and release their products into the interstitial fluid. The interstitial fluid cannot, however, be considered a large reservoir for nutrients or a large sink for metabolic products, because its volume is less than half that of the cells that it serves. The well-being of individual cells therefore depends heavily on the homeostatic mechanisms that regulate the composition of the interstitial fluid. This task is accomplished by continuously exposing the interstitial fluid to "fresh" circulating plasma fluid.

As blood passes through capillaries, solutes exchange between plasma and interstitial fluid by the process of diffusion. The net result of transcapillary diffusion is always that the interstitial fluid tends to take on the composition of the incoming blood. If, for example, potassium ion concentration in the interstitium of a particular skeletal muscle was higher than that in the plasma entering the muscle, then potassium would diffuse into the blood as it passes through the muscle's capillaries. Since this removes potassium from the interstitial fluid, its potassium ion concentration would decrease. It would stop decreasing when the net movement of potassium into capillaries no longer occurs, that is, when the concentration of the interstitial fluid reaches that of incoming plasma.

Three conditions are essential for this circulatory mechanism to effectively control the composition of the interstitial fluid: (1) there must be adequate blood flow through the tissue capillaries, (2) the chemical composition of the incoming (or arterial) blood must be controlled to be that which is optimal in the interstitial fluid, and (3) diffusion distances must be short. Figure 1–1 shows how the cardiovascular transport system operates to accomplish these tasks. As discussed earlier, substances are transported between cells and plasma in capillary vessels within organs by the process of diffusion. This transport occurs over extremely small distances because no cell in the body is located farther than approximately 10 μm from a capillary. Over such microscopic distances, *diffusion* is a very rapid process that can move huge quantities of material. Diffusion, however, is a very poor mechanism for moving substances from the capillaries of one organ, such as the lungs, to the capillaries of another organ that may be 1 m or more distant. Consequently, substances are transported between organs by the process of *convection*, by which the substances easily move along with blood flow because they are either dissolved or contained within blood. The relative distances involved in cardiovascular transport are not well illustrated in Figure 1–1. If the figure were drawn to scale, with 1 inch representing the distance from capillaries to cells within a calf muscle, then the capillaries in the lungs would have to be located about 15 miles away!

The overall functional arrangement of the cardiovascular system is illustrated in Figure 1–2. Since a functional rather than an anatomical viewpoint is expressed in this figure, the role of heart appears in three places: as the right heart pump, as the left heart pump, and as the heart muscle tissue. It is common practice to view the cardiovascular system as (1) the *pulmonary circulation*, composed of the right heart

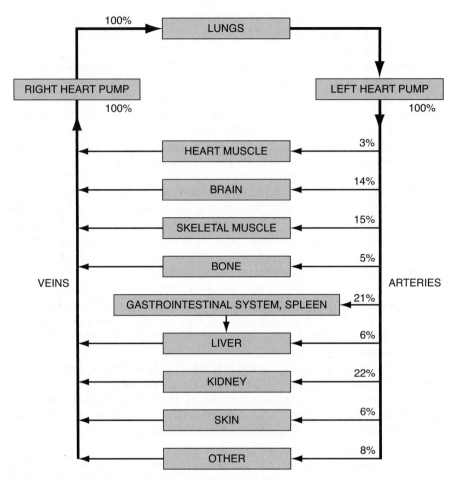

Figure 1–2. Cardiovascular circuitry, indicating the percentage distribution of cardiac output to various organ systems in a resting individual.

pump and the lungs, and (2) the *systemic circulation*, in which the left heart pump supplies blood to the systemic organs (all structures except the gas exchange portion of the lungs). The pulmonary and systemic circulations are arranged in series, that is, one after the other. Consequently, both the right and left hearts must pump an identical volume of blood per minute. This amount is called the *cardiac output*. A cardiac output of 5 to 6 L/min is normal for a resting individual.

As indicated in Figure 1–2, the systemic organs are functionally arranged in parallel (ie, side by side) within the cardiovascular system. There are two important consequences of this parallel arrangement. First, nearly all systemic organs receive blood of identical composition—that which has just left the lungs and is known as *arterial blood*. Second, the flow through any one of the systemic organs can be controlled independently of the flow through the other organs. Thus, for example, the cardiovascular response to whole body exercise can involve increased blood flow through some organs, decreased blood flow through others, and unchanged blood flow through yet others.

Many of the organs in the body help perform the task of continually reconditioning the blood circulating in the cardiovascular system. Key roles are played by organs, such as the lungs, that communicate with the external environment. As is evident from the arrangement shown in Figure 1–2, any blood that has just passed through a systemic organ returns to the right heart and is pumped through the lungs, where oxygen and carbon dioxide are exchanged. Thus, the blood's gas composition is always reconditioned immediately after leaving a systemic organ.

Like the lungs, many of the systemic organs also serve to recondition the composition of blood, although the flow circuitry precludes their doing so each time the blood completes one circuit. The kidneys, for example, continually adjust the electrolyte composition of the blood passing through them. Because the blood conditioned by the kidneys mixes freely with all the circulating blood and because electrolytes and water freely pass through most capillary walls, the kidneys control the electrolyte balance of the entire internal environment. To achieve this, it is necessary that a given unit of blood pass often through the kidneys. In fact, the kidneys (under resting conditions) normally receive about one-fifth of the cardiac output. This greatly exceeds the amount of flow that is necessary to supply the nutrient needs of the renal tissue. This situation is common to organs that have a blood-conditioning function.

Blood-conditioning organs can also withstand, at least temporarily, severe reductions of blood flow. Skin, for example, can easily tolerate a large reduction in blood flow when it is necessary to conserve body heat. Most of the large abdominal organs also fall into this category. The reason is simply that because of their blood-conditioning functions, their normal blood flow is far in excess of that necessary to maintain their basal metabolic needs.

The brain, heart muscle, and skeletal muscles typify organs in which blood flows solely to supply the metabolic needs of the tissue. They do not recondition the blood for the benefit of any other organ. Normally, the blood flow to the brain and the heart muscle is only slightly greater than that required for their metabolism; hence, they do not tolerate blood flow interruptions well. Unconsciousness can occur within a few seconds after stoppage of cerebral flow, and permanent brain damage can occur in as little as 4 minutes without flow. Similarly, the heart muscle (myocardium) normally consumes approximately 75% of the oxygen supplied to it, and the heart's pumping ability begins to deteriorate within beats of a coronary flow interruption. As we shall see later, the task of providing adequate blood flow to the brain and the heart muscle receives a high priority in the overall operation of the cardiovascular system.

THE BASIC PHYSICS OF BLOOD FLOW

As outlined above, the task of maintaining interstitial homeostasis requires that an adequate quantity of blood flow continuously through each of the millions of capillaries in the body. In a resting individual, this adds up to a cardiac output

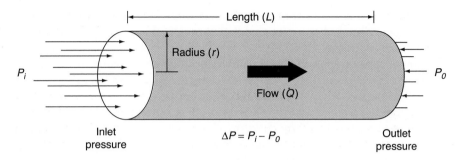

Figure 1–3. Factors influencing fluid flow through a tube.

of approximately 5 L/min (about 80 gallons/h). As people go about their daily lives, the metabolic rates and therefore the blood flow requirements in different organs and regions throughout the body change from moment to moment. Thus, the cardiovascular system must continuously adjust both the magnitude of cardiac output and how that cardiac output is distributed to different parts of the body. One of the most important keys to comprehending how the cardiovascular system operates is a thorough understanding of the relationship among the physical factors that determine the rate of fluid flow through a tube.

② The tube depicted in Figure 1–3 might represent a segment of any vessel in the body. It has a certain length (L) and a certain internal radius (r) through which blood flows. Fluid flows through the tube only when the pressures in the fluid at the inlet and outlet ends (P_i and P_o) are unequal, that is, when there is a pressure difference (ΔP) between the ends. Pressure differences supply the driving force for flow. Because friction develops between the moving fluid and the stationary walls of a tube, vessels tend to resist fluid movement through them. This *vascular resistance* is a measure of how difficult it is to make fluid flow through the tube, that is, how much of a pressure difference it takes to cause a certain flow. The all-important relationship among flow, pressure difference, and resistance is described by the *basic flow equation* as follows:

$$\text{Flow} = \frac{\text{pressure difference}}{\text{resistance}}$$

$$\dot{Q} = \frac{\Delta P}{R}$$

where $\dot{Q}$ = flow rate (volume/time)
  ΔP = pressure difference (mmHg[1])
  R = resistance to flow (mmHg × time/volume)

---

[1] Although pressure is most correctly expressed in units of force per unit area, it is customary to express pressures within the cardiovascular system in millimeters of mercury. For example, mean arterial pressure may be said to be 100 mmHg because it is same as the pressure existing at the bottom of a mercury column 100 mm high. All cardiovascular pressures are expressed relative to atmospheric pressure, which is approximately 760 mmHg.

The basic flow equation may be applied not only to a single tube but also to complex networks of tubes, for example, the vascular bed of an organ or the entire systemic system. The flow through the brain, for example, is determined by the difference in pressure between cerebral arteries and veins divided by the overall resistance to flow through the vessels in the cerebral vascular bed. It should be evident from the basic flow equation that there are only two ways in which blood flow through any organ can be changed: (1) by changing the pressure difference across its vascular bed or (2) by changing its vascular resistance. Most often, it is changes in an organ's vascular resistance that cause the flow through the organ to change.

From the work of the French physician Jean Leonard Marie Poiseuille (1799–1869), who performed experiments on fluid flow through small glass capillary tubes, it is known that the resistance to flow through a cylindrical tube depends on several factors, including the radius and length of the tube and the viscosity of the fluid flowing through it. These factors influence resistance to flow as follows:

$$R = \frac{8L\eta}{\pi r^4}$$

where r = internal radius of the tube
L = tube length
η = fluid viscosity (Greek letter "*eta*")

Note that the internal radius of the tube is raised to the fourth power in this equation. Thus, even small changes in the internal radius of a tube have a very large influence on its resistance to flow. For example, halving the inside radius of a tube will increase its resistance to flow by 16-fold.

The preceding equations may be combined into one expression known as the *Poiseuille equation*, which includes all the terms that influence flow through a cylindrical vessel.[2]

$$\dot{Q} = \Delta P \frac{\pi r^4}{8L\eta}$$

Again, note that flow occurs only when a pressure difference exists. It is not surprising then that arterial blood pressure is an extremely important and carefully regulated cardiovascular variable. Also note once again that for any given pressure difference, tube radius has a very large influence on the flow through a tube. It is logical, therefore, that organ blood flows are regulated primarily through changes in the radius of vessels within organs. Although vessel length and blood viscosity

---

[2] Poiseuille's equation properly applies only to a homogeneous fluid flowing through rigid nontapered tubes with a certain flow pattern called *laminar flow*. Although not all these conditions are rigidly met for any vessel within the body, the approximation is close enough to permit general conclusions to be drawn from Poiseuille's equation.

are factors that influence vascular resistance, they are not variables that can be easily manipulated for the purpose of moment-to-moment control of blood flow.

In regard to the overall cardiovascular system as depicted in Figures 1–1 and 1–2, one can conclude that blood flows through the vessels within an organ only because a pressure difference exists between the blood in the arteries supplying the organ and the veins draining it. The primary job of the heart pump is to keep the pressure within arteries higher than that within veins. Normally, the average pressure in systemic arteries is near 100 mmHg, and the average pressure in systemic veins is near 0 mmHg.

Therefore, because the pressure difference (ΔP) is identical across all systemic organs, cardiac output is distributed among the various systemic organs solely on the basis of their individual resistances to flow. Because blood flows along the path of least resistance, organs with relatively low resistance receive relatively high flow.

THE HEART

Pumping Action

The heart lies in the center of the thoracic cavity and is suspended by its attachments to the great vessels within a thin fibrous sac called the *pericardium*. A small amount of fluid in the sac lubricates the surface of the heart and allows it to move freely during contraction and relaxation. Blood flow through all organs is passive and occurs only because arterial pressure is kept higher than venous pressure by the pumping action of the heart. The right heart pump provides the energy necessary to move blood through the pulmonary vessels, and the left heart pump provides the energy to move blood through the systemic organs.

The amount of blood pumped per minute from each ventricle (the *cardiac output*, CO) depends on the volume of blood ejected per beat (the *stroke volume*, SV) and the number of heartbeats per minute (the *heart rate*, HR) as follows:

$$CO = SV \times HR$$
$$\text{volume/minute} = \text{volume/beat} \times \text{beats/minute}$$

It should be evident from this relationship that all influences on cardiac output must act by changing either the heart rate or the stroke volume. These influences will be described in detail in subsequent chapters.

The pathway of blood flow through the chambers of the heart is indicated in Figure 1–4. Venous blood returns from the systemic organs to the right atrium via the superior and inferior venae cavae. It then passes through the *tricuspid valve* into the right ventricle and from there is pumped through the *pulmonic valve* into the pulmonary circulation via the pulmonary arteries. Oxygenated pulmonary venous blood flows in pulmonary veins to the left atrium and passes through the *mitral valve* into the left ventricle. From there it is pumped through the *aortic valve* into the aorta to be distributed to the systemic organs.

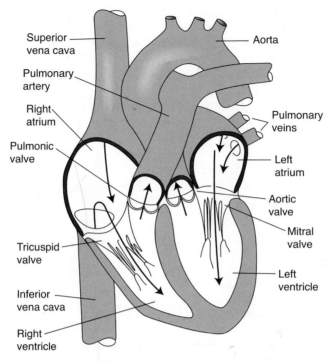

Figure 1–4. Pathway of blood flow through the heart.

Although the gross anatomy of the right heart pump is somewhat different from that of the left heart pump, the pumping principles are identical. Each pump consists of a ventricle, which is a closed chamber surrounded by a muscular wall, as illustrated in Figure 1–5. The valves are structurally designed to allow flow in only one direction and passively open and close in response to the direction of the pressure differences across them. Ventricular pumping action occurs because the volume of the intraventricular chamber is cyclically changed by rhythmic and synchronized contraction and relaxation of the individual cardiac muscle cells that lie in a circumferential orientation within the ventricular wall.

When the ventricular muscle cells are contracting, they generate a circumferential tension in the ventricular walls that causes the pressure within the chamber to increase. As soon as the ventricular pressure exceeds the pressure in the pulmonary artery (right pump) or aorta (left pump), blood is forced out of the chamber through the outlet valve as shown in Figure 1–5. This phase of the cardiac cycle during which the ventricular muscle cells are contracting is called *systole*. Because the pressure is higher in the ventricle than in the atrium during systole, the inlet or atrioventricular (AV) valve is closed. When the ventricular muscle cells relax, the pressure in the ventricle falls below that in the atrium, the AV valve opens, and the ventricle refills with blood, as shown on the right side in Figure 1–5. This portion of the cardiac cycle is called *diastole*. The outlet valve is closed during diastole because arterial pressure is

VENTRICULAR SYSTOLE   VENTRICULAR DIASTOLE

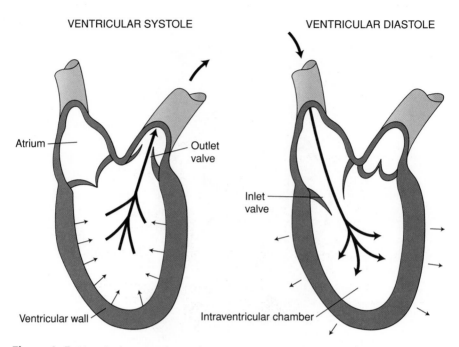

Atrium ─── ─── Outlet valve

Inlet ─── valve

Ventricular wall ─── Intraventricular chamber ───

Figure 1–5. Ventricular pumping action.

greater than intraventricular pressure. After the period of diastolic filling, the systolic phase of a new cardiac cycle is initiated.

Excitation

Efficient pumping action of the heart requires a precise coordination of the contraction of millions of individual cardiac muscle cells. Contraction of each cell is triggered when an electrical excitatory impulse (*action potential*) sweeps over its membrane. Proper coordination of the contractile activity of the individual cardiac muscle cells is achieved primarily by the conduction of action potentials from one cell to the next via gap junctions that connect all cells of the heart into a functional syncytium (ie, acting as one synchronous unit). In addition, muscle cells in certain areas of the heart are specifically adapted to control the frequency of cardiac excitation, the pathway of conduction, and the rate of the impulse propagation through various regions of the heart. The major components of this specialized excitation and conduction system are shown in Figure 1–6. These include the *sinoatrial node* (SA node), the *atrioventricular node* (AV node), the *bundle of His,* and the right and left *bundle branches* made up of specialized cells called *Purkinje* fibers.

The SA node contains specialized cells that normally function as the heart's pacemaker and initiate the action potential that is conducted through the heart. The

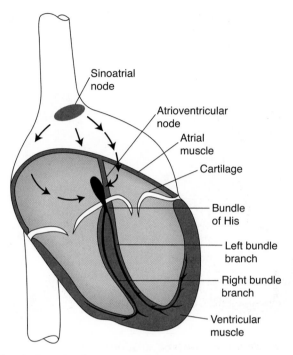

Figure 1–6. Electrical conduction system of the heart.

AV node contains slowly conducting cells that normally function to create a slight delay between atrial contraction and ventricular contraction. The Purkinje fibers are specialized for rapid conduction and ensure that all ventricular cells contract at nearly the same instant.

Requirements for Effective Operation

For effective, efficient ventricular pumping action, the heart must be functioning properly in five basic respects:

1. The contractions of individual cardiac muscle cells must occur at regular intervals and be synchronized (not *arrhythmic*).
2. The valves must open fully (not *stenotic*).
3. The valves must not leak (not *insufficient* or *regurgitant*).
4. The muscle contractions must be forceful (not *failing*).
5. The ventricles must fill adequately during diastole.

In the subsequent chapters, we will study in detail how these requirements are met in the normal heart.

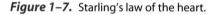

Ventricular end-diastolic volume

Figure 1–7. Starling's law of the heart.

Control of the Heart and Cardiac Output

DIASTOLIC FILLING

One of the most fundamental causes of variations in stroke volume was described by William Howell in 1884 and by Otto Frank in 1894 and formally stated by E. H. Starling in 1918. These investigators demonstrated that as cardiac filling increases during diastole, the volume ejected during systole also increases. As a consequence, and as illustrated in Figure 1–7, with other factors being equal, stroke volume increases as cardiac end-diastolic volume increases. This phenomenon (commonly referred to as Starling's law of the heart) is an intrinsic property of the cardiac muscle and is one of the primary regulators of cardiac output. The mechanisms responsible for this phenomenon depend largely on the cardiac muscle cells' length–tension relationship and will be described in detail in subsequent chapters.

Autonomic Neural Influences

Although the heart can inherently beat on its own, cardiac function can be influenced profoundly by neural inputs from both the sympathetic and parasympathetic divisions of the autonomic nervous system. These inputs allow us to modify cardiac pumping as is appropriate to meet changing homeostatic needs of the body. All portions of the heart are richly innervated by *adrenergic sympathetic fibers.* When active, these sympathetic nerves release *norepinephrine* (noradrenaline) on cardiac cells. Norepinephrine interacts with β_1-adrenergic receptors on cardiac muscle cells to increase the heart rate, increase the action potential conduction velocity, and increase the force of contraction and rates of contraction and relaxation. Overall, sympathetic activation acts to increase cardiac pumping.

Cholinergic parasympathetic nerve fibers travel to the heart via the vagus nerve and innervate the SA node, the AV node, and the atrial muscle. When active, these parasympathetic nerves release *acetylcholine* on cardiac muscle cells. Acetylcholine interacts with *muscarinic* receptors on cardiac muscle cells to decrease the heart rate (SA node) and decrease the action potential conduction velocity (AV node). Parasympathetic nerves may also act to decrease the force of contraction of atrial (not ventricular) muscle cells. Overall, parasympathetic activation acts to decrease cardiac pumping. Usually, an increase in parasympathetic nerve activity is accompanied by a decrease in sympathetic nerve activity, and vice versa.

THE VASCULATURE

Blood that is ejected into the aorta by the left heart passes consecutively through many different types of vessels before it returns to the right heart. As illustrated in Figure 1–8, the major vessel classifications are *arteries, arterioles, capillaries, venules,*

	ARTERIES		ARTERIOLES	CAPILLARIES	VENULES		VEINS	
	Aorta							Venae cavae
Internal diameter	2.5 cm	0.4 cm	30 μm	5 μm	70 μm	0.5 cm	3 cm
Wall thickness	2 mm	1 mm	20 μm	1 μm	7 μm	0.5 mm	1.5 mm
Number	1	160	5×10^7	10^{10}	10^8	200	2
Total cross-sectional area	4.5 cm^2	20 cm^2	400 cm^2	4500 cm^2	4000 cm^2	40 cm^2	18 cm^2

Figure 1–8. Structural characteristics of the peripheral vascular system.

and *veins*. These consecutive vascular segments are distinguished from one another by differences in their physical dimensions, morphological characteristics, and function. One thing that all these vessels have in common is that they are lined with a contiguous single layer of endothelial cells. In fact, this is true for the entire circulatory system including the heart chambers and even the valve leaflets.

Some representative physical characteristics of these major vessel types are shown in Figure 1–8. It should be realized, however, that the vascular bed is a continuum and that the transition from one type of vascular segment to another does not occur abruptly. The total cross-sectional area through which blood flows at any particular level in the vascular system is equal to the sum of the cross-sectional areas of all the individual vessels arranged in parallel at that level. The number and total cross-sectional area values presented in Figure 1–8 are estimates for the entire systemic circulation.

Arteries are thick-walled vessels that contain, in addition to some smooth muscle, a large component of elastin and collagen fibers. Primarily because of the elastin fibers, which can stretch to twice their unloaded length, arteries can expand to accept and temporarily store some of the blood ejected by the heart during systole and then, by passive recoil, supply this blood to the organs downstream during diastole. The aorta is the largest artery and has an internal (lumenal) diameter of approximately 25 mm. Arterial diameter decreases with each consecutive branching, and the smallest arteries have diameters of approximately 0.1 mm. The consecutive arterial branching pattern causes an exponential increase in arterial numbers. Thus, although individual vessels get progressively smaller, the total cross-sectional area available for blood flow within the arterial system increases to severalfold that in the aorta. Arteries are often referred to as *conduit* vessels because they have relatively low and unchanging resistance to flow.

Arterioles are smaller and structured differently than arteries. In proportion to lumen size, arterioles have much thicker walls with more smooth muscle and less elastic material than do arteries. Because arterioles are so muscular, their diameters can be actively changed to regulate the blood flow through peripheral organs. Despite their minute size, arterioles are so numerous that in parallel their collective cross-sectional area is much larger than that at any level in arteries. Arterioles are often referred to as *resistance* vessels because of their high and changeable resistance, which regulates peripheral blood flow through individual organs.

Capillaries are the smallest vessels in the vasculature. In fact, red blood cells with diameters of 7 μm must deform to pass through them. The capillary wall consists of a single layer of endothelial cells that separate the blood from the interstitial fluid by only approximately 1 μm. Capillaries contain no smooth muscle and thus lack the ability to change their diameters actively. They are so numerous that the total collective cross-sectional area of all the capillaries in systemic organs is more than 1000 times that of the root of the aorta. Given that capillaries are approximately 0.5 mm in length, the total surface area available for exchange of material between blood and interstitial fluid can be calculated; it exceeds 100 m^2. For obvious reasons, capillaries are viewed as the *exchange* vessels of the cardiovascular system. In addition to the transcapillary diffusion of solutes that occurs across these vessel walls, there can sometimes be net movements of fluid (volume) into and/or out of capillaries. For example, tissue swelling (*edema*) is a result of net fluid movement from plasma into the interstitial space.

After leaving capillaries, blood is collected in venules and veins and returned to the heart. Venous vessels have very thin walls in proportion to their diameters. Their walls contain smooth muscle, and their diameters can actively change. Because of their thin walls, venous vessels are quite distensible. Therefore, their diameters change passively in response to small changes in transmural distending pressure (ie, the difference between the internal and external pressures across the vessel wall). Venous vessels, especially the larger ones, also have one-way valves that prevent reverse flow. As will be discussed later, these valves are especially important in the cardiovascular system's operation during standing and during exercise. It turns out that peripheral venules and veins normally contain more than 50% of the total blood volume. Consequently, they are commonly thought of as the *capacitance* vessels. More importantly, *changes* in venous volume greatly influence cardiac filling and therefore cardiac pumping. Thus, peripheral veins actually play an extremely important role in controlling cardiac output.

Control of Blood Vessels

 Blood flow through individual vascular beds is profoundly influenced by changes in the activity of sympathetic nerves innervating arterioles. These nerves release norepinephrine at their endings that interacts with α-*adrenergic* receptors on the smooth muscle cells to cause contraction and thus arteriolar constriction. The reduction in arteriolar diameter increases vascular resistance and decreases blood flow. These neural fibers provide the most important means of *reflex* control of vascular resistance and organ blood flow.

Arteriolar smooth muscle is also very responsive to changes in the local chemical conditions within an organ that accompany changes in the metabolic rate of the organ. For reasons to be discussed later, increased tissue metabolic rate leads to arteriolar dilation and increased tissue blood flow.

Venules and veins are also richly innervated by sympathetic nerves and constrict when these nerves are activated. The mechanism is the same as that involved with arterioles. Thus, increased sympathetic nerve activity is accompanied by decreased venous volume. The importance of this phenomenon is that venous constriction tends to increase cardiac filling and therefore cardiac output via Starling's law of the heart.

There is no important neural or local metabolic control of either arterial or capillary vessels.

BLOOD

 Blood is a complex fluid that serves as the medium for transporting substances between the tissues of the body and performs a host of other functions as well. Normally, approximately 40% of the volume of whole blood is occupied by blood cells that are suspended in the watery fluid, *plasma*, which accounts for the rest of the volume. The fraction of blood volume occupied by cells is termed as the *hematocrit*, a clinically important parameter.

$$\text{Hematocrit} = \text{cell volume/total blood volume}$$

Blood Cells

Blood contains three general types of "formed elements": red cells, white cells, and platelets (see Appendix A). All are formed in bone marrow from a common stem cell. Red cells are by far the most abundant. They are specialized to carry oxygen from the lungs to other tissues by binding oxygen to *hemoglobin*, an iron-containing heme protein concentrated within red blood cells. Because of the presence of hemoglobin, blood can transport 40 to 50 times the amount of oxygen that plasma alone could carry. In addition, the hydrogen ion buffering capacity of hemoglobin is vitally important to the blood's capacity to transport carbon dioxide.

A small, but important, fraction of the cells in blood is white cells or *leukocytes*. Leukocytes are involved in immune processes. Appendix A gives more information on the types and function of leukocytes. Platelets are small cell fragments that are important in the blood-clotting process.

Plasma

Plasma is the liquid component of blood and, as indicated in Appendix B, is a complex solution of electrolytes and proteins. *Serum* is the fluid obtained from a blood sample after it has been allowed to clot. For all practical purposes, the composition of serum is identical to that of plasma except that it contains none of the clotting proteins.

Inorganic *electrolytes* (inorganic ions such as sodium, potassium, chloride, and bicarbonate) are the most concentrated solutes in plasma. Of these, sodium and chloride are by far the most abundant and, therefore, are primarily responsible for plasma's normal osmolarity of about 300 mOsm/L. To a first approximation, the "stock" of the plasma soup is a 150-mM solution of sodium chloride. Such a solution is called "isotonic saline" and has many clinical uses as a fluid that is compatible with cells.

Plasma normally contains many different *proteins*. Most plasma proteins can be classified as *albumins*, *globulins*, or *fibrinogen* on the basis of different physical and chemical characteristics used to separate them. More than 100 distinct plasma proteins have been identified and each presumably serves some specific function. Many plasma proteins are involved in blood clotting or immune/defense reactions. Many others are important carrier proteins for a variety of substances including fatty acids, iron, copper, vitamin D, and certain hormones.

Proteins do not readily cross capillary walls and, in general, their plasma concentrations are much higher than their concentrations in the interstitial fluid. As will be discussed, plasma proteins play an important osmotic role in transcapillary fluid movement and consequently in the distribution of extracellular volume between the plasma and interstitial compartments. *Albumin* plays an especially strong role in this regard simply because it is by far the most abundant of the plasma proteins.

Plasma also serves as the vehicle for transporting nutrients and waste products. Thus, a plasma sample contains many small organic molecules such as glucose, amino acids, urea, creatinine, and uric acid whose measured values are useful in clinical diagnosis.

FOUNDATION FOR SUBSEQUENT CHAPTERS

This first chapter has presented an overall description of the design of the cardiovascular system. Some important, basic, bottom-line principles that should help you understand many aspects of cardiovascular function have been included. (See the study questions at the end of this chapter, for example.)

Subsequent chapters will expand these concepts in much greater detail, but we urge students not to lose sight of the overall picture presented in this chapter. It may be useful to repeatedly refer back to this material.

KEY CONCEPTS

 The primary role of the cardiovascular system is to maintain homeostasis in the interstitial fluid.

 The physical law that governs cardiovascular operation is that flow through any segment is equal to pressure difference across that segment divided by its resistance to flow; ie, $\dot{Q} = \Delta P/R$.

 The heart pumps blood by rhythmically filling and ejecting blood from the ventricular chambers that are served by passive one-way inlet and outlet valves.

 Changes in heart rate and stroke volume (and therefore cardiac output) can be accomplished by alterations in ventricular filling and by alterations in autonomic nerve activity to the heart.

 Blood flow through individual organs is regulated by changes in the diameter of their arterioles.

 Changes in arteriolar diameter can be accomplished by alterations in sympathetic nerve activity and by variations in local conditions.

 Blood is a complex suspension of red cells, white cells, and platelets in plasma that is ideally suited to carry gases, salts, nutrients, and waste molecules throughout the system.

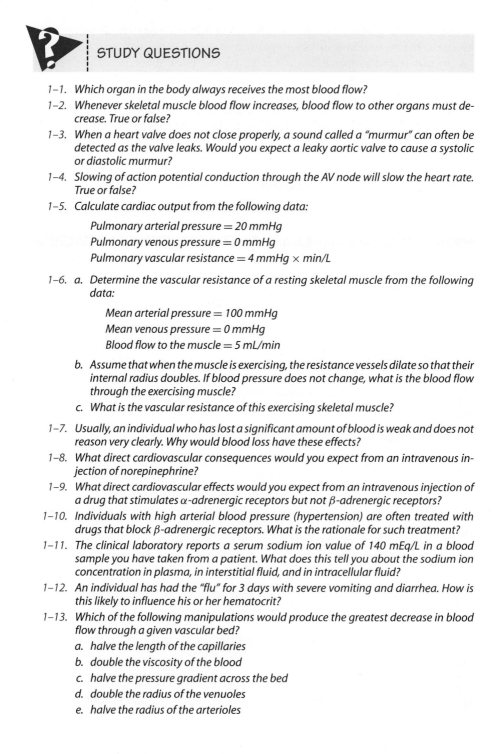

STUDY QUESTIONS

1–1. Which organ in the body always receives the most blood flow?

1–2. Whenever skeletal muscle blood flow increases, blood flow to other organs must decrease. True or false?

1–3. When a heart valve does not close properly, a sound called a "murmur" can often be detected as the valve leaks. Would you expect a leaky aortic valve to cause a systolic or diastolic murmur?

1–4. Slowing of action potential conduction through the AV node will slow the heart rate. True or false?

1–5. Calculate cardiac output from the following data:

> Pulmonary arterial pressure = 20 mmHg
> Pulmonary venous pressure = 0 mmHg
> Pulmonary vascular resistance = 4 mmHg × min/L

1–6. a. Determine the vascular resistance of a resting skeletal muscle from the following data:

> Mean arterial pressure = 100 mmHg
> Mean venous pressure = 0 mmHg
> Blood flow to the muscle = 5 mL/min

  b. Assume that when the muscle is exercising, the resistance vessels dilate so that their internal radius doubles. If blood pressure does not change, what is the blood flow through the exercising muscle?

  c. What is the vascular resistance of this exercising skeletal muscle?

1–7. Usually, an individual who has lost a significant amount of blood is weak and does not reason very clearly. Why would blood loss have these effects?

1–8. What direct cardiovascular consequences would you expect from an intravenous injection of norepinephrine?

1–9. What direct cardiovascular effects would you expect from an intravenous injection of a drug that stimulates α-adrenergic receptors but not β-adrenergic receptors?

1–10. Individuals with high arterial blood pressure (hypertension) are often treated with drugs that block β-adrenergic receptors. What is the rationale for such treatment?

1–11. The clinical laboratory reports a serum sodium ion value of 140 mEq/L in a blood sample you have taken from a patient. What does this tell you about the sodium ion concentration in plasma, in interstitial fluid, and in intracellular fluid?

1–12. An individual has had the "flu" for 3 days with severe vomiting and diarrhea. How is this likely to influence his or her hematocrit?

1–13. Which of the following manipulations would produce the greatest decrease in blood flow through a given vascular bed?

  a. halve the length of the capillaries

  b. double the viscosity of the blood

  c. halve the pressure gradient across the bed

  d. double the radius of the venuoles

  e. halve the radius of the arterioles

1-14. *Arteries play which of the following functional roles in the systemic vascular system?*
  a. *as conduit vessels*
  b. *as capacitance vessels*
  c. *as resistance vessels*
  d. *as exchange vessels*

1-15. *You need to determine the correct dose of an IV drug that distributes only within the extracellular space. Which of the following values would be the closest estimate of the extracellular fluid volume of a healthy young adult male weighing 100 kg (220 lb)?*
  a. *3 L*
  b. *5 L*
  c. *8 L*
  d. *10 L*
  e. *20 L*

Characteristics of
Cardiac Muscle Cells

2

OBJECTIVES

The student understands the ionic basis of the spontaneous electrical activity of cardiac muscle cells:

▶ *Describes how membrane potentials are created across semipermeable membranes by transmembrane ion concentration differences.*

▶ *Defines equilibrium potential and knows its normal value for potassium and sodium ions.*

▶ *States how membrane potential reflects a membrane's relative permeability to various ions.*

▶ *Defines resting potential and action potential.*

▶ *Describes the characteristics of "fast" and "slow" response action potentials.*

▶ *Identifies the refractory periods of the cardiac cell electrical cycle.*

▶ *Defines threshold potential and describes the interaction between ion channel conditions and membrane potential during the depolarization phase of the action potential.*

▶ *Defines pacemaker potential and describes the basis for rhythmic electrical activity of cardiac cells.*

▶ *Lists the phases of the cardiac cell electrical cycle and states the membrane's permeability alterations responsible for each phase.*

The student knows the normal process of cardiac electrical excitation:

▶ *Describes gap junctions and their role in cardiac excitation.*

▶ *Describes the normal pathway of action potential conduction through the heart.*

▶ *Indicates the timing at which various areas of the heart are electrically excited and identifies the characteristic action potential shapes and conduction velocities in each major part of the conduction system.*

▶ *States the relationship between electrical events of cardiac excitation and the P, QRS, and T waves, the PR interval, and the ST segment of the electrocardiogram.*

The student understands the factors that control the heart rate and action potential conduction in the heart:

▶ *States how diastolic potentials of pacemaker cells can be altered to produce changes in the heart rate.*

▶ *Describes how cardiac sympathetic and parasympathetic nerves alter the heart rate and conduction of cardiac action potentials.*

▶ *Defines the terms* chronotropic *and* dromotropic.

The student understands the contractile processes of cardiac muscle cells:
▶ *Lists the subcellular structures responsible for cardiac muscle cell contraction.*
▶ *Defines and describes the* excitation–contraction *process.*
▶ *Defines* isometric, isotonic, *and* afterloaded *contractions of the cardiac muscle.*
▶ *Identifies the influence of altered preload on the tension producing and shortening capabilities of the cardiac muscle.*
▶ *Describes the influence of altered afterload on the shortening capabilities of the cardiac muscle.*
▶ *Defines the terms* contractility *and* inotropic state *and describes the influence of altered contractility on the tension producing and shortening capabilities of the cardiac muscle.*
▶ *Describes the effect of altered sympathetic neural activity on the cardiac inotropic state.*
▶ *States the relationships between ventricular volume and muscle length, between intraventricular pressure and muscle tension and the law of Laplace.*

Cardiac muscle cells are responsible for providing the power to drive blood through the circulatory system. Coordination of their activity depends on an electrical stimulus that is regularly initiated at an appropriate rate and reliably conducted through the entire heart. Mechanical pumping action depends on a robust contraction of the muscle cells that results in repeating cycles of tension development, shortening and relaxation. In addition, mechanisms to adjust the excitation and contraction characteristics must be available to meet the changing demands of the circulatory system. This chapter focuses on these electrical and mechanical properties of cardiac muscle cells that underlie normal heart function.

ELECTRICAL ACTIVITY OF CARDIAC MUSCLE CELLS

In all striated muscle cells, contraction is triggered by a rapid voltage change called an *action potential* that occurs on the cell membrane. Cardiac muscle cell action potentials differ sharply from those of skeletal muscle cells in three important ways that promote synchronous rhythmic excitation of the heart: (1) they can be self-generating; (2) they can be conducted directly from cell to cell; and (3) they have long duration, which precludes fusion of individual twitch contractions. To understand these special electrical properties of the cardiac muscle and how cardiac function depends on them, the basic electrical properties of excitable cell membranes must first be reviewed.

Membrane Potentials

All cells have an electrical potential (voltage) across their membranes. Such *membrane potentials* are caused by a separation of electrical charges across the membrane itself. The only way that the membrane potential can change is for electrical charges to move across (ie, current to flow through) the cell membrane.

There are two important corollaries to this statement: (1) the rate of change of membrane voltage is directly proportional to the net current across the membrane and (2) membrane voltage is stable (ie, unchanging) only when there is no net current across the membrane.

Unlike a wire, current across cell membranes is not carried by electrons but by the movement of ions through the cell membrane. The three ions that are the most important determinants of cardiac membrane potentials are sodium (Na^+) and calcium (Ca^{2+}), which are more concentrated in the interstitial fluid than they are inside cells, and potassium (K^+), which is more concentrated in intracellular than interstitial fluid. In general, such ions are very insoluble in lipids. Consequently, they cannot pass into or out of a cell through the lipid bilayer of the membrane itself. Instead, these ions cross the membrane only via various protein structures that are embedded in and span across the lipid cell wall. There are three general types of such transmembrane protein structures that are involved in ion movement across the cell membrane: (1) ion *channels*, (2) ion *exchangers*, and (3) ion *pumps*.[1] All are very specific for particular ions. For example, a "sodium channel" is a transmembrane protein structure that allows only Na^+ ions to pass into or out of a cell according to the net electrochemical forces acting on Na^+ ions.

The subsequent discussion concentrates on ion channel operation because ion channels (as opposed to transporters and pumps) are responsible for the resting membrane potential and for the rapid changes in membrane potential that constitute the cardiac cell action potential. Ion channels are under complex control and can be "opened," "closed," or "inactivated." The net result of the status of membrane channels to a particular ion is commonly referred to as the membrane's *permeability* to that ion. For example, "high permeability to sodium" implies that many of the Na^+ ion channels are in their open state at that instant. Precise timing of the status of ion channels accounts for the characteristic membrane potential changes that occur when cardiac cells are activated.

Figure 2–1 shows how ion concentration differences can generate an electrical potential across the cell membrane. Consider first, as shown at the top of this figure, a cell that (1) has K^+ more concentrated inside the cell than outside, (2) is permeable only to K^+ (ie, only K^+ channels are open), and (3) has no initial transmembrane potential. Because of the concentration difference, K^+ ions (positive charges) will diffuse out of the cell. Meanwhile, negative charges, such as protein anions, cannot leave the cell because the membrane is impermeable to them. Thus, the K^+ efflux will make the cytoplasm just inside the cell membrane more electrically negative (deficient in positively charged ions) and at the same time make the interstitial fluid just outside the cell membrane more electrically positive (rich in positively charged ions). Now K^+ ion, being positively charged, is attracted to regions of electrical negativity. Therefore, when K^+ diffuses out of a cell, it creates an electrical potential

---

[1] "Channels" can be thought of as passive ion-specific holes in the membrane through which a particular ion will move according to the electrochemical forces acting on it. "Exchangers" are passive devices that couple the movement of two or more specific ions across the membrane according to the collective net electrochemical forces acting on all the ions involved. "Pumps" use the chemical energy of splitting ATP to move ions across the cell membrane against prevailing electrochemical forces.

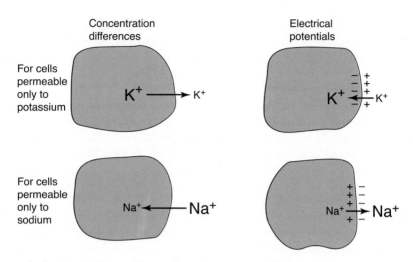

Figure 2–1. Electrochemical basis of membrane potentials.

across the membrane that tends to attract it back into the cell. There exists one membrane potential called the *potassium equilibrium potential* at which the electrical forces tending to pull K⁺ into the cell exactly balance the concentration forces tending to drive K⁺ out. When the membrane potential has this value, there is no *net* movement of K⁺ across the membrane. With the normal concentrations of approximately 145 m*M* K⁺ inside cells and 4 m*M* K⁺ in the extracellular fluid, the K⁺ equilibrium potential is roughly −90 mV (more negative inside than outside by nine-hundredths of a volt).[2] A membrane that is permeable only to K⁺ will inherently and rapidly (essentially instantaneously) develop the potassium equilibrium potential. In addition, membrane potential changes require the movement of so few ions that concentration differences are not significantly affected by the process.

As depicted in the bottom half of Figure 2–1, similar reasoning shows how a membrane permeable only to Na⁺ would have the *sodium equilibrium potential* across it. The sodium equilibrium potential is approximately +70 mV, with the normal extracellular Na⁺ concentration of 140 m*M* and intracellular Na⁺ concentration of 10 m*M*. Real cell membranes, however, are never permeable to just Na⁺ or just K⁺. When a membrane is permeable to both of these ions, the membrane potential will lie somewhere between the Na⁺ equilibrium potential and the K⁺ equilibrium potential. Just what membrane potential will exist at any instant depends on the relative permeability of the membrane to Na⁺ and K⁺. The more permeable the membrane is to K⁺ than to Na⁺, the closer the membrane potential will be to −90 mV. Conversely, when the permeability to Na⁺ is high relative to the

---

[2] The equilibrium potential (E_{eq}) for any ion (X^z) is determined by its intracellular and extracellular concentrations as indicated in the Nernst equation:

$$E_{eq} = \frac{-61.5\,\text{mV}}{z} \log_{10} \frac{[X^z]\text{inside}}{[X^z]\text{outside}}$$

permeability to K^+, the membrane potential will be closer to $+70$ mV.[3] A *stable* membrane potential that lies between the sodium and potassium equilibrium potentials implies that there is no *net* current across the membrane. This situation may well be the result of opposite but balanced sodium and potassium currents across the membrane.

Because of low or unchanging permeability or low concentration, roles played by ions other than Na^+ and K^+ in determining membrane potential are usually minor and often ignored. However, as discussed later, calcium ions (Ca^{2+}) do participate in the cardiac muscle action potential. Like Na^+, Ca^{2+} is more concentrated outside cells than inside. The equilibrium potential for Ca^{2+} is approximately $+100$ mV, and the cell membrane tends to become more positive on the inside when the membrane's permeability to Ca^{2+} rises.

Under resting conditions, most heart muscle cells have membrane potentials that are quite close to the potassium equilibrium potential. Thus, both electrical and concentration gradients favor Na^+ and Ca^{2+} entry into the resting cell. However, the very low permeability of the resting membrane to Na^+ and Ca^{2+}, in combination with an energy-requiring sodium pump that extrudes Na^+ from the cell, prevents Na^+ and Ca^{2+} from gradually accumulating inside the resting cell.[4,5]

Cardiac Cell Action Potentials

 Action potentials of cells from different regions of the heart are not identical but have varying characteristics that are important to the overall process of cardiac excitation.

Some cells within a specialized conduction system have the ability to act as pacemakers and to spontaneously initiate action potentials, whereas ordinary cardiac muscle cells do not (except under unusual conditions). Basic membrane electrical features of an ordinary cardiac muscle cell and a cardiac pacemaker-type cell are shown in Figure 2–2. Action potentials from these cell types are referred to as "fast-response" and "slow-response" action potentials, respectively. As shown in Figure 2–2A, fast-response action potentials are characterized by a rapid depolarization (phase 0) with a substantial overshoot (positive inside voltage), a rapid reversal of the overshoot potential (phase 1), a long plateau (phase 2), and a repolarization (phase 3) to a stable, high (ie, large negative) resting membrane potential (phase 4). In comparison, the slow-response action potentials are characterized by a slower initial depolarization phase, a lower amplitude overshoot,

---

[3] A quantitative description of how Na^+ and K^+ concentrations and the relative permeability (P_{Na}/P_K) to these ions affect membrane potential (E_m) is given by the following equation:

$$E_m = -61.5\,\text{mV}\log_{10}\left(\frac{[K^+]_i + P_{Na}/P_K[Na^+]_i}{[K^+]_o + P_{Na}/P_K[Na^+]_o}\right)$$

[4] The sodium pump not only removes Na^+ from the cell but also pumps K^+ into the cell. Because more Na^+ is pumped out than K^+ is pumped in (3:2), the pump is said to be electrogenic. The resting membrane potential becomes slightly less negative than normal when the pump is abruptly inhibited.

[5] The steep sodium gradient also promotes Ca^{2+} removal from the cytoplasm via a sodium/calcium exchanger.

Figure 2-2. Time course of membrane potential (A and B) and ion permeability changes (C and D) that occur during "fast-response" (*left*) and "slow-response" (*right*) action potentials.

a shorter and less stable plateau phase, and a repolarization to an unstable, slowly depolarizing "resting" potential (Figure 2–2B). The unstable resting potential seen in pacemaker cells with slow-response action potentials is variously referred to as *phase 4 depolarization, diastolic depolarization,* or *pacemaker potential.* Such cells are usually found in the sinoatrial (SA) and atrioventricular (AV) nodes.

As indicated at the bottom of Figure 2–2A, cells are in an absolute refractory state during most of the action potential (ie, they cannot be stimulated to fire another action potential). Near the end of the action potential, the membrane is relatively refractory and can be reexcited only by a larger than normal stimulus. Immediately after the action potential, the membrane is transiently hyperexcitable and is said to be in a "vulnerable" or "supranormal" period. Similar alterations in membrane excitability occur during slow action potentials but at present are not well characterized.

Recall that the membrane potential of any cell at any given instant depends on the relative permeability of the cell membrane to specific ions. As in all excitable cells, cardiac cell *action* potentials are the result of transient changes in the ionic permeability of the cell membrane that are triggered by an initial depolarization. Figures 2–2C and 2–2D indicate the changes in the membrane's permeabilities to K^+, Na^+, and Ca^{2+} that produce the various phases of the fast- and slow-response action potentials.[6] Note that during the resting phase, the membranes of both types of cells are more permeable to K^+ than to Na^+ or Ca^{2+}. Therefore, the membrane potentials are close to the potassium equilibrium potential (of -90 mV) during this period. In pacemaker-type cells, at least three mechanisms are thought to contribute to the slow depolarization of the membrane observed during the diastolic interval. First, there is a progressive decrease in the membrane's permeability to K^+ during the resting phase, and second, the permeability to Na^+ increases slightly. The gradual increase in the Na^+/K^+ permeability ratio will cause the membrane potential to move slowly away from the K^+ equilibrium potential (-90 mV) in the direction of the Na^+ equilibrium potential. Third, there is a slight increase in the permeability of the membrane to calcium ions, which results in an inward movement of these positively charged ions and also contributes to the diastolic depolarization.

When the membrane potential depolarizes to a certain *threshold* potential in either type of cell, major rapid alterations in the permeability of the membrane to specific ions are triggered. Once initiated, these permeability changes cannot be stopped and they proceed to completion.

The characteristic rapid rising phase of the fast-response action potential is a result of a sudden increase in Na^+ permeability. This produces what is referred to as the *fast inward current* of Na^+ and causes the membrane potential to move rapidly toward the sodium equilibrium potential. As indicated in Figure 2–2C, this period of very high sodium permeability (phase 0) is short-lived.[7] Development and maintenance of a depolarized *plateau* state (phase 2) is accomplished by the interactions of at least three separate processes: (1) a sustained reduction in K^+ permeability, (2) a slowly developed and sustained increase in the membrane's permeability to Ca^{2+}, and (3) electrogenic action of an Na^+/Ca^{2+} exchanger in which three Na^+ ions move into the cell in exchange for a single Ca^{2+} ion moving out of the cell.

The initial fast inward current is small (or even absent) in cells that have slow-response action potentials. The slow rising phase of these action potentials is therefore primarily a result of an inward movement of Ca^{2+} ions. In both types of cells,

---

[6] The membrane's permeability to a particular ion is not synonymous with the transmembrane current of that ion. The transmembrane current of any ion is the product of the membrane's permeability to it times the electrochemical driving forces acting on it. For example, the resting membrane is quite permeable to K^+ but there is little net K^+ movement because the resting membrane potential is very close to the potassium equilibrium potential.

[7] This is followed by a very brief increase in potassium permeability (not shown in Figure 2–2C) that allows a brief outward going potassium current (i_{To}) that contributes to the early repolarization (phase 1).

the membrane is repolarized (phase 3) to its original resting potential as the K^+ permeability increases and the Ca^{2+} and Na^+ permeabilities return to their low resting values. These late permeability changes produce what is referred to as the *delayed outward current.*

The overall smoothly graded permeability changes that produce action potentials are the net result of alterations in each of the many individual ion channels within the plasma membrane of a single cell.[8] These ion channels are generally made up of very long polypeptide chains that loop repeatedly across the cell membrane. These loops form a hollow channel between the intra- and extracellular fluids that are structurally quite specific for certain ions. The open/closed status of the channels can be altered by configurational changes in parts of the molecules within the channel ("gates") so that when open, ions move down their electrochemical gradient either into or out of the cell (high permeability). It is a largely unsolved mystery as to what specific mechanisms control the operation of these channels and cause the timing of their operation to so stereotypically follow the onset of a cardiac action potential. Some of the current thinking about these processes is presented later. Certain types of channels are called *voltage-gated channels* (or voltage-operated channels) because their probability of being open varies with membrane potential. Other types of channels, called *ligand-gated channels* (or receptor-operated channels), are activated by certain neurotransmitters or other specific signal molecules. Table 2–1 lists some of the major currents and channel types involved in cardiac cell electrical activity.

Some of the voltage-gated channels respond to a sudden onset, sustained change in membrane potential by only a brief period of activation. However, changes in membrane potential of slower onset but the same magnitude may fail to activate these channels at all. To explain such behavior, it is postulated that these channels have two independently operating "gates"—an *activation gate* and an *inactivation gate*—both of which must be open for the channel as a whole to be open. Both these gates respond to changes in membrane potential but do so with different voltage sensitivities and time courses.

These concepts are illustrated in Figure 2–3. In the resting state, with the membrane polarized to near −80 mV, the activation or *m* gate of the fast Na^+ channel is closed, but its inactivation or *h* gate is open (Figure 2–3A). With a rapid depolarization of the membrane to threshold, the Na^+ channels will be activated strongly to allow an inrush of positive sodium ions that further depolarizes the membrane and thus initiates a "fast" response action potential as illustrated in Figure 2–3B. This occurs because the *m* gate responds to membrane depolarization by opening more quickly than the *h* gate responds by closing. Thus, a rapid depolarization to threshold is followed by a brief, but strong, period of Na^+ channel activation wherein the *m* gate is open but the *h* gate has yet to close.

---

[8] The experimental technique of *patch clamping* has made it possible to study the operation of individual ion channels. The patch clamp data indicate that a single channel is either open or closed at any instant in time; there are no graded states of partial opening. What is graded is the percentage of time that a given channel spends in the open state, and the total number of channels that are currently in the open state.

Table 2–1. Characteristics of Important Cardiac Ion Channels in Order of Their Participation in an Action Potential

Current	Channel	Gating mechanism	Functional role
i_{K1}	K$^+$ channel (inward rectifier)	Voltage	Maintains high K$^+$ permeability during phase 4 Its decay contributes to diastolic depolarization Its suppression during phases 0 to 2 contributes to plateau
i_{Na}	Na$^+$ channel (fast)	Voltage	Accounts for phase 0 of action potential Inactivation may contribute to phase 1 of action potential
i_{To}	K$^+$ channel (transient outward)	Voltage	Contributes to phase 1 of action potential
i_{Ca}	Ca^{2+} channel (slow inward, L channels)	Both	Contributes to phase 2 of action potential Inactivation may contribute to phase 3 of action potential Is enhanced by sympathetic stimulation and β-adrenergic agents
i_K	K$^+$ channel (delayed rectifier)	Voltage	Causes phase 3 of action potential Is enhanced by increased intracellular Ca^{2+}
i_{KATP}	K$^+$ channel (ATP-sensitive)		Increases K$^+$ permeability when [ATP] is low
i_{KACh}	K$^+$ channel (acetylcholine-activated)	Ligand	Responsible for effects of vagal stimulation Decreases diastolic depolarization (and the heart rate) Hyperpolarizes resting membrane potential Shortens phase 2 of the action potential
i_f ("funny")	Na$^+$ (pacemaker current)	Both	Is activated by hyperpolarization and contributes to the diastolic depolarization Is enhanced by sympathetic stimulation and β-adrenergic agents Is suppressed by vagal stimulation

The initial membrane depolarization also causes the activation (*d*) gate of the Ca^{2+} channel to open after a brief delay. This permits the slow inward current of Ca^{2+} ions, which helps maintain the depolarization through the plateau phase of the action potential (Figure 2–3C). Ultimately, repolarization occurs because of both a delayed inactivation of the Ca^{2+} channel (by closure of the *f* gates) and an opening of K$^+$ channels (which are not shown in Figure 2–3). Multiple

Figure 2–3. A conceptual model of cardiac membrane ion channels: at rest (**A**), during the initial phases of the fast-response (**B** and **C**), and the slow-response action potentials (**D** and **E**).

factors influence the operation of K^+ channels. For example, high intracellular Ca^{2+} concentration contributes to activation of K^+ channels during repolarization. The h gates of sodium channels remain closed during the remainder of the action potential, effectively inactivating the Na^+ channel and contributing to the long cardiac refractory period, which lasts until the end of phase 3. With repolarization, both gates of the sodium channel return to their original position and the channel is now ready to be reactivated by a subsequent depolarization.

The slow-response action potential shown in the right half of Figure 2–3 differs from the fast-response action potential primarily because of the lack of a strong activation of the fast Na^+ channel at its onset. This is a direct consequence of a slow depolarization to the threshold potential. Slow depolarization gives the inactivating *h* gates time to close even as the activating *m* gates are opening (Figure 2–3D). Thus, in a slow-response action potential, there is no initial period where all the sodium channels of a cell are essentially open at once. The depolarization beyond threshold is slow and caused primarily by the influx of Ca^{2+} through slow channels (Figure 2–3E).

Although cells in certain areas of the heart typically have fast-type action potentials and cells in other areas normally have slow-type action potentials, it is important to recognize that all cardiac cells are potentially capable of having either type of action potential, depending on how fast they depolarize to the threshold potential. As we shall see, rapid depolarization to the threshold potential is usually an event forced on a cell by the occurrence of an action potential in an adjacent cell. Slow depolarization to threshold occurs when a cell itself spontaneously and gradually loses its resting polarization, which normally happens only in the SA node. A *chronic* moderate depolarization of the resting membrane (caused, for example, by moderately high extracellular K^+ concentration) can inactivate the fast channels (by closing the *h* gates) without inactivating the slow Ca^{2+} channels. Under these conditions, all cardiac cell action potentials will be of the slow type. Large, sustained depolarizations, however, can inactivate both the fast and slow channels and thus make the cardiac muscle cells completely inexcitable.

Conduction of Cardiac Action Potentials

Action potentials are conducted over the surface of individual cells because active depolarization in any one area of the membrane produces local currents in the intracellular and extracellular fluids that passively depolarize immediately adjacent areas of the membrane to their voltage threshold for active depolarization.

In the heart, cardiac muscle cells are connected end-to-end by structures called *intercalated disks*. These disks contain the following: (1) *firm mechanical attachments* between adjacent cell membranes by proteins called *adherins* in structures called *desmosomes* and (2) *low-resistance electrical connections* between adjacent cells through channels formed by proteins called *connexin* in structures called *gap junctions*. Figure 2–4 shows schematically how these gap junctions allow action potential propagation from cell to cell.

Cells B, C, and D are shown in the resting phase with more negative charges inside than outside. Cell A is shown in the plateau phase of an action potential and has more positive charges inside than outside. Because of the gap junctions, electrostatic attraction can cause a local current flow (ion movement) between the depolarized membrane of active cell A and the polarized membrane of resting cell B, as indicated

How do SA nodal cells
Spontaneously depolarize?
- atrial pressure?

Resting cell C

Cell A with action potential

Resting cell B

Resting cell D

Gap junction (nexus)

Figure 2–4. Local currents and cell-to-cell conduction of cardiac muscle cell action potentials.

by the arrows in the figure. This ion movement depolarizes the membrane of cell B. Once the local currents from active cell A depolarize the membrane of cell B near the gap junction to the threshold level, an action potential will be triggered at that site and will be conducted over cell B. Because cell B branches (a common morphological characteristic of cardiac muscle fibers), its action potential will evoke action potentials on cells C and D. This process is continued through the entire myocardium. Thus, an action potential initiated at *any* site in the myocardium will be conducted from cell to cell throughout the entire myocardium.

The speed at which an action potential propagates through a region of cardiac tissue is called the *conduction velocity*. The conduction velocity varies considerably in different areas in the heart and is determined by three variables. First, conduction velocity is directly dependent on the diameter of the muscle fiber involved. Thus, conduction over small-diameter cells in the AV node is significantly slower than conduction over large-diameter cells in the ventricular Purkinje system. Second, conduction velocity is also directly dependent on the intensity of the local depolarizing currents, which are in turn directly determined by the rate of rise of the action potential. Rapid depolarization favors rapid conduction. Third, conduction velocity is dependent on the capacitive and/or resistive properties of the cell membranes, gap junctions, and cytoplasm. Electrical characteristics of gap junctions can be influenced by external conditions that promote phosphorylation/dephosphorylation of the connexin proteins.

Details of the overall consequences of the cardiac conduction system are shown in Figure 2–5. As noted earlier, the specific electrical adaptations of various cells in the heart are reflected in the characteristic shape of their action potentials that are shown in the right half of Figure 2–5. Note that the action potentials shown in Figure 2–5 have been positioned to indicate the time when the electrical impulse that originates in the SA node reaches other areas of the heart. Cells of the SA node act as the heart's normal pacemaker and determine the heart rate. This is because the spontaneous depolarization of the resting membrane is most rapid in SA nodal cells, and they reach their threshold potential before cells elsewhere.

The action potential initiated by an SA nodal cell first spreads progressively through the atrial wall. Action potentials from cells in two different regions of the

via Bachmann's Bundle

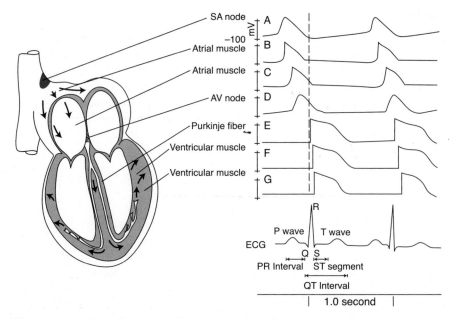

Figure 2–5. Electrical activity of the heart: single-cell voltage recordings (traces A to G) and lead II electrocardiogram.

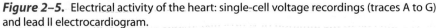

atria are shown in Figure 2–5: one close to the SA node and one more distant from the SA node. Both cells have similarly shaped action potentials, but their temporal displacement reflects the fact that it takes some time for the impulse to spread over the atria. As shown in Figure 2–5, action potential conduction is greatly slowed as it passes through the AV node. This is because of the small size of the AV nodal cells and the slow rate of rise of their action potentials. Since the AV node delays the transfer of the cardiac excitation from the atria to the ventricles, atrial contraction can contribute to ventricular filling just before the ventricles contract. Note also that AV nodal cells have a faster spontaneous depolarization during the resting period than other cells of the heart except those of the SA node. The AV node is sometimes referred to as a latent pacemaker, and in many pathological situations it (rather than the SA node) controls the heart rhythm.

Because of sharply rising action potentials and other factors, such as large cell diameters, electrical conduction is extremely rapid in Purkinje fibers. This allows the Purkinje system to transfer the cardiac impulse to cells in many areas of the ventricle nearly in unison. Action potentials from muscle cells in two areas of the ventricle are shown in Figure 2–5. Because of the high conduction velocity in ventricular tissue, there is only a small discrepancy in their time of onset. Note in Figure 2–5 that the ventricular cells which are the last to depolarize have shorter duration action potentials and thus are the first to repolarize. The physiological importance of this unexpected behavior is not clear, but it does have an influence on the electrocardiograms that is discussed in Chapter 4.

Electrocardiograms

Fields of electrical potential caused by the electrical activity of the heart extend through the extracellular fluid of the body and can be measured with electrodes placed on the body surface. *Electrocardiography* provides a record of how the voltage between two points on the body surface changes with time as a result of the electrical events of the cardiac cycle. At any instant of the cardiac cycle, the electrocardiogram indicates the net electrical field that is the summation of many weak electrical fields being produced by voltage changes occurring on individual cardiac cells at that instant. When a large number of cells are simultaneously depolarizing or repolarizing, large voltages are observed on the electrocardiogram. Because the electrical impulse spreads through the heart tissue in a consistent pathway, the temporal pattern of voltage change recorded between two points on the body surface is also consistent and will repeat itself with each heart cycle.

The lower trace of Figure 2–5 represents a typical recording of the voltage changes normally measured between the right arm and the left leg as the heart goes through two cycles of electrical excitation; this record is called a lead II electrocardiogram and is discussed in detail in Chapter 4. The major features of an electrocardiogram are the *P wave,* the PR interval, the *QRS complex,* the QT interval, and the *T wave.* The P wave corresponds to atrial depolarization; the PR interval to the conduction time through the atria and AV node: the QRS complex, to ventricular depolarization; the QT interval to the duration of ventricular systole and the T wave, to ventricular repolarization.

Control of Heart Beating Rate

Normal rhythmic contractions of the heart occur because of spontaneous electrical pacemaker activity (automaticity) of cells in the SA node. The interval between heartbeats (and thus the heart rate) is determined by how long it takes the membranes of these pacemaker cells to spontaneously depolarize to the threshold level. The SA nodal cells fire at a spontaneous or *intrinsic rate* (≈ 100 beats per minute) in the absence of any outside influences. Outside influences *are* required, however, to increase or decrease automaticity from its intrinsic level.

The two most important outside influences on automaticity of SA nodal cells come from the autonomic nervous system. Fibers from both the sympathetic and parasympathetic divisions of the autonomic system terminate on cells in the SA node, and these fibers can modify the intrinsic heart rate. Activating the cardiac sympathetic nerves (increasing cardiac sympathetic *tone*) increases the heart rate. Increasing the cardiac parasympathetic tone slows the heart rate. As shown in Figure 2–6, both the parasympathetic and sympathetic nerves influence the heart rate by altering the course of spontaneous depolarization of the resting potential in SA pacemaker cells.

Cardiac parasympathetic fibers, which travel to the heart through the *vagus* nerves, release the transmitter substance *acetylcholine* on SA nodal cells. Acetylcholine increases the permeability of the resting membrane to K^+ and decreases the diastolic

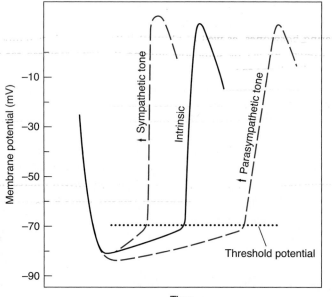

Figure 2–6. The effect of sympathetic and parasympathetic tone on pacemaker potential.

permeability to Na^+.[9] As indicated in Figure 2–6, these permeability changes have two effects on the resting potential of cardiac pacemaker cells: (1) they cause an initial hyperpolarization of the resting membrane potential by bringing it closer to the K^+ equilibrium potential and (2) they slow the rate of spontaneous depolarization of the resting membrane. Both of these effects increase the time between beats by prolonging the time required for the resting membrane to depolarize to the threshold level. Because there is normally some continuous *tonic* activity of cardiac parasympathetic nerves, the normal resting heart rate is approximately 70 beats per minute.

Sympathetic nerves release the transmitter substance *norepinephrine* on cardiac cells. In addition to other effects discussed later, norepinephrine acts on SA nodal cells to increase the inward currents carried by Na^+ (i_f) and by Ca^{2+} during the diastolic interval.[10] These changes will increase the heart rate by increasing the rate of diastolic depolarization as shown in Figure 2–6.

---

[9] Acetylcholine interacts with muscarinic receptors on the SA nodal cell membrane that in turn are linked to inhibitory G proteins, G_i. The activation of G_i has two effects: (1) an increase in K^+ conductance resulting from an increased opening of the K_{Ach} channels and (2) a suppression of adenylate cyclase leading to a fall in intracellular cyclic adenosine monophosphate, which reduces the inward-going pacemaker current carried by Na^+ (i_f).

[10] Norepinephrine interacts with β_1-adrenergic receptors on the SA nodal cell membrane that in turn are linked to stimulatory G proteins, G_s. The activation of G_s increases adenylate cyclase, leading to an increase in intracellular cyclic AMP that increases the open-state probability of the pacemaker Na^+ current channel (i_f).

In addition to sympathetic and parasympathetic nerves, there are many (usually less important) factors that can alter the heart rate. These include a number of ions and circulating hormones, as well as physical influences such as temperature and atrial wall stretch. All act by somehow altering the time required for the resting membrane to depolarize to the threshold potential. An abnormally high concentration of Ca^{2+} in the extracellular fluid, for example, tends to decrease the heart rate by shifting the threshold potential. Factors that increase the heart rate are said to have a *positive chronotropic effect.* Those that decrease the heart rate have a *negative chronotropic effect.*

Besides their effect on the heart rate, autonomic fibers also influence the conduction velocity of action potentials through the heart. Increases in sympathetic activity increase conduction velocity (have a *positive dromotropic effect*), whereas increases in parasympathetic activity decrease conduction velocity (have a *negative dromotropic effect*). These effects are most notable at the AV node and can influence the duration of the PR interval.

MECHANICAL ACTIVITY OF THE HEART

Cardiac Muscle Contraction

Contraction of the cardiac muscle cell is initiated by the action potential signal acting on intracellular organelles to evoke tension generation and/or shortening of the cell. In this section, we describe (1) the subcellular processes involved in coupling the excitation to the contraction of the cell (EC coupling) and (2) the mechanical properties of cardiac cells.

Basic histological features of cardiac muscle cells are quite similar to those of skeletal muscle cells and include (1) an extensive myofibrillar structure made up of parallel interdigitating thick and thin filaments arranged in serial units called *sarcomeres*, which are responsible for the mechanical processes of shortening and tension development[11]; (2) a complex internal compartmentation of the cytoplasm by an intracellular membrane system called the *sarcoplasmic reticulum* (SR), which sequesters calcium during the diastolic interval with the help of the calcium-storage protein *calsequestrin*; (3) regularly spaced, extensive invaginations of the cell

---

[11] Proteins making up the thick and thin filaments are collectively referred to as "contractile proteins." The *thick filament* consists of a protein called *myosin*, which has a long straight tail with two globular heads each of which contains an ATP-binding site and an actin-binding site; light chains are loosely associated with the heads and their phosphorylation may regulate (or modulate) muscle function. The *thin filament* consists of several proteins including *actin*—two α-helical strands of polymerized subunits (g-actin) with sites that interact with the heads of myosin molecules to form cross-bridges with the thick filaments; *tropomyosin*—a regulatory fibrous-type protein lying in the groove of the actin α-helix, which prevents actin from interacting with myosin when the muscle is at rest; and *troponin*—a regulatory protein consisting of three subunits: *troponin C*, which binds calcium ions during activation and initiates the configurational changes in the regulatory proteins that expose the actin site for cross-bridge formation; *troponin T*, which anchors the troponin complex to tropomyosin; and *troponin I*, which participates in the inhibition of actin–myosin interaction at rest. In addition, the macromolecule, *titin*, extends from the Z disk to the M line and contributes significantly to the passive stiffness of cardiac muscle over its normal working range.

membrane (sarcolemma), called *T tubules*, which appear to be connected to parts of the SR ("junctional" SR) by dense strands ("feet") and which carry the action potential signal to the inner parts of the cell; and (4) a large number of mitochondria that provide the oxidative phosphorylation pathways needed to ensure a ready supply of adenosine triphosphate (ATP) to meet the high metabolic needs of the cardiac muscle. Students are encouraged to consult a histology textbook for specific cellular, morphological details.

Excitation–Contraction Coupling

Muscle action potentials trigger mechanical contraction through a process called *excitation–contraction coupling,* which is illustrated in Figure 2–7. The major event of excitation–contraction coupling is a dramatic rise in the intracellular free Ca^{2+} concentration. The "resting" intracellular free Ca^{2+} concentration is less than 0.1 μM. In contrast, during maximum activation of the contractile apparatus, the intracellular free Ca^{2+} concentration reaches nearly 100 μM. When the wave of depolarization passes over the muscle cell membrane and down the T tubules, Ca^{2+} is released from the SR into the intracellular fluid.

Figure 2–7. Excitation–contraction coupling and sarcomere shortening.

As indicated on the left side of Figure 2–7, the specific trigger for this release appears to be the entry of calcium into the cell via the L-type calcium channels and an increase in Ca^{2+} concentration in the region just under the sarcolemma on the surface of the cell and throughout the t-tubular system. Unlike the skeletal muscle, this highly localized increase in calcium is essential for triggering the massive release of calcium from the SR. This *calcium-induced calcium release* is a result of opening calcium-sensitive release channels on the SR.[12] Although the amount of Ca^{2+} that enters the cell during a single action potential is quite small compared with that released from the SR, it is essential not only for triggering the SR calcium release but also for maintaining adequate levels of Ca^{2+} in the intracellular stores over the long run.

When the intracellular Ca^{2+} level is high (>1.0 μM), links called *cross-bridges* form between two types of filaments found within the muscle. Sarcomere units, as depicted in the lower part of Figure 2–7, are joined end to end at Z lines to form *myofibrils*, which run the length of the muscle cell. During contraction, thick and thin filaments slide past one another to shorten each sarcomere and thus the muscle as a whole. The bridges form when the regularly spaced myosin heads from thick filaments attach to regularly spaced sites on the actin molecules in the thin filaments. Subsequent deformation of the bridges results in a pulling of the actin molecules toward the center of the sarcomere. This actin–myosin interaction requires energy from ATP. In resting muscles, the attachment of myosin to the actin sites is inhibited by troponin and tropomyosin. Calcium causes muscle contraction by interacting with troponin C to cause a configurational change that removes the inhibition of the actin sites on the thin filament. Because a single cross-bridge is a very short structure, gross muscle shortening requires that cross-bridges repetitively form, produce incremental movement between the myofilaments, detach, form again at a new actin site, and so on in a cyclic manner.

There are several processes that participate in the reduction of intracellular Ca^{2+} that terminates the contraction. These processes are illustrated on the right side of Figure 2–7. Approximately 80% of the calcium is actively taken back up into the SR by the action of Ca^{2+}-ATPase pumps located in the network part of the SR.[13] About 20% of the calcium is extruded from the cell into the extracellular fluid either via the Na^{+}–Ca^{2+} exchanger located in the sarcolemma[14] or via sarcolemmal Ca^{2+}-ATPase pumps.

---

[12] These channels may be blocked by the plant alkaloid ryanodine and are activated by the methylxanthine caffeine. These agents are chemical tools used to assess properties of these SR channels.

[13] The action of these pumps is regulated by the protein phospholamban. When this protein is phosphorylated (eg, by the action of norepinephrine), the rate of Ca^{2+} resequestration is increased and the rate of relaxation is enhanced. *faster you relax ; faster you can get another A.P.*

[14] The Na^{+}–Ca^{2+} exchanger is powered by the sodium gradient across the sarcolemma, which, in turn, is maintained by the Na^{+}/K^{+}-ATPase. This exchanger is electrogenic in that three Na^{+} ions move into the cell in exchange for each Ca^{2+} ion that moves out. This net inward movement of positive charge may contribute to the maintenance of the plateau phase of the action potential. The cardiac glycoside, digitalis, slows down the Na^{+}/K^{+} pump and thus reduces the sodium gradient, which, in turn, results in an increase in intracellular Ca^{2+}. This mechanism contributes to the positive effect of cardiac glycosides on the contractile force of the failing heart.

Excitation–contraction coupling in the cardiac muscle is different from that in the skeletal muscle in that it may be modulated; different intensities of actin–myosin interaction (contraction) can result from a single action potential trigger in the cardiac muscle. The mechanism for this is largely dependent on variations in the amount of Ca^{2+} reaching the myofilaments and therefore the number of cross-bridges activated during the twitch. This ability of the cardiac muscle to vary its contractile strength—that is, change its *contractility*—is extremely important to cardiac function, as discussed in a later section of this chapter.

The duration of the cardiac muscle cell contraction is approximately the same as that of its action potential. Therefore, the electrical refractory period of a cardiac muscle cell is not over until the mechanical response is completed. As a consequence, heart muscle cells cannot be activated rapidly enough to cause a fused (tetanic) state of prolonged contraction. This is fortunate because intermittent contraction and relaxation are essential for the heart's pumping action.

Electrical activity precedes mechanical activity.

Cardiac Muscle Cell Mechanics

The cross-bridge interaction that occurs after a muscle is activated to contract gives the muscle the potential to develop force and/or shorten. Whether it does one, the other, or some combination of the two depends primarily on what is allowed to happen by the external constraints placed on the muscle during the contraction. For example, activating a muscle whose ends are held rigidly causes it to develop tension, but it cannot shorten. This is called an *isometric* ("fixed length") contraction. The force that a muscle produces during an isometric contraction indicates its maximum ability to develop tension. At the other extreme, activating an unrestrained muscle causes it to shorten without force development because it has nothing to develop force against. This type of contraction is called an *isotonic* ("fixed tension") contraction. Under such conditions, a muscle shortens with its maximum possible velocity (called V_{max}), which is determined by the maximum possible rate of cross-bridge cycling. Adding load to the muscle decreases the velocity and extent of its shortening. Thus, the course of a muscle contraction depends on both the inherent capabilities of the muscle and the external constraints placed on the muscle during contraction. Muscle cells in the ventricular wall operate under different constraints during different phases of each cardiac cycle. To understand ventricular function, the manner in which the cardiac muscle behaves when constrained in several different ways must first be examined.

fixed length

Isometric Contractions: Length–Tension Relationships

The influence of muscle length on the behavior of the cardiac muscle during isometric contraction is illustrated in Figure 2–8. The top panel shows the experimental arrangement for measuring muscle force at rest and during contraction at three different lengths. The middle panel shows time records of muscle tensions recorded at each of the three lengths in response to an external stimulus, and the bottom panel shows a graph of the resting and peak tension results plotted against muscle length.

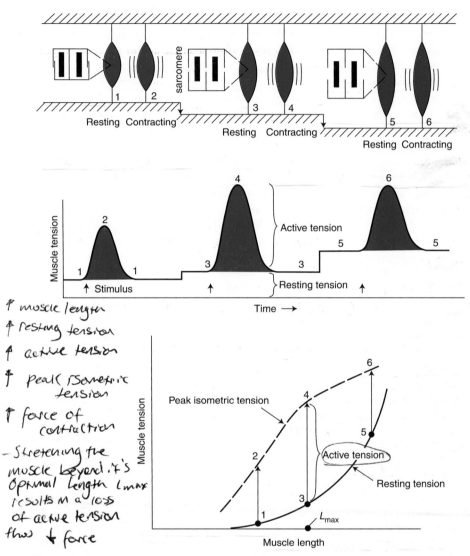

(handwritten margin notes:)
↑ muscle length
↑ resting tension
↑ active tension
↑ peak isometric tension
↑ force of contraction
- Stretching the muscle beyond it's optimal length L_{max} results in a loss of active tension thus ↓ force

Figure 2–8. Isometric contractions and the effect of muscle length on resting tension and active tension development.

The first important fact illustrated in Figure 2–8 is that force is required to stretch a resting muscle to different lengths. This force is called the *resting tension*. The lower curve in the graph in Figure 2–8 shows the resting tension measured at different muscle lengths and is referred to as the *resting length–tension curve*. When a muscle is stimulated to contract while its length is held constant, it develops an additional component of tension called *active* or *developed tension*. The *total tension* exerted by a muscle during contraction is the sum of the active and resting tensions.

Isometric L-T Relationship

1. Optimal L → optimal active tension
2. ↑Resting tension → ↑ isometric tension
3. Crossbridge Proximity; Ca Sensitivity
4. ↑resting L → ↑ [Ca] intracellular

The second important fact illustrated in Figure 2–8 is that the active tension developed by the cardiac muscle during the course of an isometric contraction depends very much on the muscle length at which the contraction occurs. Active tension development is maximum at some intermediate length referred to as L_{max}. Little active tension is developed at very short or very long muscle lengths. Normally, the cardiac muscle operates at lengths well below L_{max} so that increasing muscle length increases the tension developed during an isometric contraction.

There are three separate mechanisms that have been proposed to explain the relationship between muscle length and developed tension. The first mechanism to be identified suggests that this relationship depends on the extent of overlap of the thick and thin filaments in the sarcomere at rest. Histological studies indicate that the changes in the resting length of the whole muscle are associated with proportional changes in the individual sarcomeres. Peak tension development occurs at sarcomere lengths of 2.2 to 2.3 μm. At sarcomere lengths shorter than approximately 2.0 μm, the opposing thin filaments may overlap or buckle and thus interfere with active tension development as shown at the top of Figure 2–8. At long sarcomere lengths, overlap may be insufficient for optimal cross-bridge formation.

Not intracellular [Ca²⁺]

The second (and perhaps more important) mechanism is based on a length-dependent change in sensitivity of the myofilaments to calcium. At short lengths only a fraction of the potential cross-bridges are apparently activated by a given increase in intracellular calcium. At longer lengths, more of the cross-bridges become activated, leading to an increase in active tension development. This change in calcium sensitivity occurs immediately after a change in length with no time delay. The "sensor" responsible for the length-dependent activation of the cardiac muscle seems to reside with the troponin C molecule, but how it happens is not fully understood.

The third mechanism rests on the observation that within several minutes after increasing the resting length of the cardiac muscle, there is an increase in the *amount* of calcium that is released with excitation, which is coupled to a further increase in force development. It is thought that stretch-sensitive ion channels in the cell membranes may be responsible for this delayed response.

To what extent each of these mechanisms is contributing to the length dependency of cardiac contractile force at any instant is neither clear nor very important in this discussion. The important point is that the dependence of active tension development on muscle length is a fundamental property of the cardiac muscle that has extremely powerful effects on heart function.

Isotonic and Afterloaded Contractions

changing length → shortening when contractile potential > load

During what is termed *isotonic* ("fixed load") contraction, a muscle shortens against a constant load. A muscle contracts isotonically when lifting a fixed weight such as the 1-g load shown in Figure 2–9. Such a 1-g weight placed on a resting muscle will result in some specific resting muscle length, which is determined by the muscle's resting length–tension curve. If the muscle were to contract isometrically at this length, it would be capable of generating a certain amount of tension, for example, 4.5 g as indicated by the dashed line in the graph in Figure 2–9. A contractile tension

Figure 2-9. Relationship of isotonic and afterloaded contractions to the cardiac muscle length–tension diagram.

of 4.5 g obviously cannot be generated while lifting a 1-g weight. When a muscle has contractile potential in excess of the tension it is actually developing, it shortens. Thus in an isotonic contraction, muscle length decreases at constant tension, as illustrated by the horizontal arrow from point 1 to point 3 in Figure 2–9. As the muscle shortens, however, its contractile potential inherently decreases, as indicated by the downward slope of the peak isometric tension curve in Figure 2–9. There exists some short length at which the muscle is capable of generating only 1 g of tension, and when this length is reached, shortening must cease.[15] Thus, the curve

---

[15] In reality, muscle shortening requires some time and the duration of a muscle twitch contraction is limited because intracellular Ca^{2+} levels are elevated only briefly following the initiation of a membrane action potential. For this and possibly other reasons, isotonic shortening may not actually proceed quite as far as the isometric tension development curve on the length–tension diagram suggests is possible. Because this complication does not alter the general correspondence between a muscle's isometric and isotonic performance, we choose to ignore it.

on the cardiac muscle length–tension diagram that indicates how much isometric tension a muscle can develop at various lengths also establishes the limit on how far muscle shortening can proceed with different loads.

Figure 2–9 also shows a complex type of muscle contraction called an *afterloaded isotonic contraction*, in which the load on the muscle at rest, the *preload*, and the load on the muscle during contraction, the *total load*, are different. In the example of Figure 2–9, the preload is equal to 1 g, and because an additional 2-g weight (the *afterload*) is engaged during contraction, the total load equals 3 g.

Because preload determines the resting muscle length, both isotonic contractions shown in Figure 2–9 begin from the same length. Because of the different loading arrangement, however, the afterloaded muscle must increase its total tension to 3 g before it can shorten. This initial tension will be developed isometrically and can be represented as going from point 1 to point 4 on the length–tension diagram. Once the muscle generates enough tension to equal the total load, its tension output is fixed at 3 g and it will now shorten isotonically because its contractile potential still exceeds its tension output. This isotonic shortening is represented as a horizontal movement on the length–tension diagram along the line from point 4 to point 5. As in any isotonic contraction, shortening must cease when the muscle's tension-producing potential is decreased sufficiently by the length change to be equal to the load on the muscle. Note that the afterloaded muscle shortens less than the non-afterloaded muscle, even though both muscles began contracting at the same initial length. The factors that affect the extent of cardiac muscle shortening during an afterloaded contraction are of special interest to us, because, as we shall see, stroke volume is determined by how far the cardiac muscle shortens under these conditions.

Afterloaded muscles shorten less than non-afterloaded even w/ initial length is constant.

Cardiac Muscle Contractility

A number of factors in addition to initial muscle length can affect the tension-generating potential of the cardiac muscle. *Any intervention that increases the peak isometric tension that a muscle can develop at a fixed length is said to increase cardiac muscle contractility.* Such an agent is said to have a *positive inotropic effect* on the heart.

The most important physiological regulator of cardiac muscle contractility is norepinephrine. When norepinephrine is released on cardiac muscle cells from sympathetic nerves, it has not only the chronotropic effect on the heart rate discussed earlier but also a pronounced, positive inotropic effect that causes cardiac muscle cells to contract more rapidly and forcefully.

The positive effect of norepinephrine on the isometric tension-generating potential is illustrated in Figure 2–10A. When norepinephrine is present in the solution bathing the cardiac muscle, the muscle will, *at every length*, develop more isometric tension when stimulated than it would in the absence of norepinephrine. In short, norepinephrine raises the peak isometric tension curve on the cardiac muscle

Handwritten annotations:
preload:
load on muscle
@ Rest

Preload
Determines
Resting Muscle
length.

tension generating
Potential is
Higher @
shorter length.

Figure 2–10. The effect of norepinephrine (NE) on isometric (**A**) and afterloaded (**B**) contractions of the cardiac muscle.

length–tension graph. Norepinephrine is said to increase cardiac muscle contractility because it enhances the forcefulness of muscle contraction *even when length is constant.* Changes in contractility and initial length can occur simultaneously, but by definition a change in *contractility* must involve a shift from one peak isometric length–tension curve to another.

Figure 2–10B shows how raising the peak isometric length–tension curve with norepinephrine increases the amount of shortening in afterloaded contractions of the cardiac muscle. With preload and total load constant, more shortening occurs in the presence of norepinephrine than in its absence. This is because when contractility is increased, the tension-generating potential is equal to the total load at a shorter muscle length. Note that norepinephrine has no effect on the resting length–tension relationship of the cardiac muscle. Thus, norepinephrine causes increased shortening by changing the final but not the initial muscle length associated with afterloaded contractions.

The cellular mechanism of the norepinephrine effect on contractility is mediated by its interaction with a β_1-adrenergic receptor. The signaling pathway involves an activation of the G_s protein–cAMP–protein kinase A, which then phosphorylates the Ca^{2+} channel, increasing the inward calcium current during the plateau of the action potential. This increase in calcium influx not only contributes to the magnitude of the rise in intracellular Ca^{2+} for a given beat but also loads the internal calcium stores, which allows more to be released during subsequent depolarizations. This increase in free Ca^{2+} during activation allows more cross-bridges to be formed and greater tension to be developed.

Because norepinephrine also causes phosphorylation of the regulatory protein, *phospholamban*, on the sarcoplasmic reticular Ca^{2+}-ATPase pump, the rate of calcium retrapping into the SR is enhanced and the rate of relaxation is increased. This is called a *positive lusitropic effect.* In addition to more rapid calcium retrapping by the SR, there is a norepinephrine-induced decrease in the action potential duration. This effect is achieved by a potassium channel alteration, occurring in response to the elevated intracellular $[Ca^{2+}]$ that increases potassium permeability, terminates the plateau phase of the action potential, and contributes to the early relaxation. Such shortening of the systolic interval is helpful in the presence of elevated heart rates that might otherwise significantly compromise diastolic filling time.

Enhanced parasympathetic activity has been shown to have a small negative inotropic effect on the heart. In the atria, where this effect is most pronounced, the negative inotropic effect is thought to be due to a shortening of the action potential and a decrease in the amount of Ca^{2+} that enters the cell during the action potential.

Changes in the heart rate also influence cardiac contractility. Recall that a small amount of extracellular Ca^{2+} enters the cell during the plateau phase of each action potential. As the heart rate increases, more Ca^{2+} enters the cells per minute. There is a buildup of intracellular Ca^{2+} and a greater amount of Ca^{2+} is released into the sarcoplasm with each action potential. Thus, a sudden increase in beating rate is followed by a progressive increase in contractile force to a higher plateau. This behavior is called the *staircase phenomenon* (or *treppe*). Changes in contractility produced by this intrinsic mechanism are sometimes referred to as *homeometric autoregulation*. The importance of such rate-dependent modulation of contractility in normal ventricular function is not clear at present.

Parasympathetic is mainly chronotropic effect

RELATING CARDIAC MUSCLE CELL MECHANICS TO VENTRICULAR FUNCTION

Certain geometric factors dictate how the length–tension relationships of cardiac muscle fibers in the ventricular wall determine the volume and pressure relationships of the ventricular chamber. The actual relationships are complex because the shape of the ventricle is complex. The ventricle is often modeled as either a cylinder or a sphere, although its actual shape lies somewhere between the

↑ HR ↑ [Ca⁺] ↑ cross bridging ↑ contractility ↑ contractile force

two. Because cardiac muscle cells are oriented circumferentially in the ventricular wall, either model can be used to illustrate three important functional points:

1. An increase in ventricular volume causes an increase in ventricular circumference and therefore an increase in the length of the individual cardiac muscle cells (and vice versa). Thus, the extent of diastolic filling of the ventricle determines the "preload." *an increase in circumference & ventricular volume*

2. At any given ventricular volume, an increase in the tension of individual cardiac muscle cells in the wall causes an increase in intraventricular pressure (and vice versa). *↑ in Intraventricular pressure ↑ wall tension*

3. As ventricular volume decreases (ie, as the ventricular radius decreases), a lesser total (collective) force is required by the muscle cells in the ventricular walls to produce any given intraventricular pressure (and vice versa). *↓ vent radius ↓ tension*
   ↑ vent radius ↑ radius more force is required; *less force required to produce pressure*

The last point is a reflection of the *law of Laplace* that states the physical relationship that must exist between total wall tension and internal pressure in any hollow vessel with circular containing walls. Regardless of whether the ventricle is envisioned as a hollow cylinder or a hollow sphere, the law of Laplace says that the *total* wall tension (T) depends on both intraventricular pressure (P) and its internal radius (r) as $T = P \times r$.

↓ T is required

One implication of the law of Laplace is that the muscle cells in the ventricular wall have a somewhat easier job of producing internal pressure at the end of ejection (when the radius is small) than at the beginning of ejection (when the radius is large). More importantly, the law of Laplace has important clinical relevance in pathological situations such as "cardiac dilation" and "cardiac hypertrophy." These are discussed in detail in Chapter 11.

The importance of all these relationships will become more apparent in the subsequent chapter as we consider how cardiac muscle cell behavior determines how the heart functions as a pump.

KEY CONCEPTS

1. *Cardiac myocyte membrane potentials are a result of the relative permeability of the membrane to various ions and their concentration differences across the membrane.*

2. *Action potentials of cardiac myocytes are a result of changes in the membrane's permeability to various ions.*

3. *Action potentials of cardiac myocytes have long plateau phases that generate long refractory periods and preclude summated or tetanic contractions.*

4. *Action potentials are spontaneously generated by pacemaker cells in the SA node and are conducted from cell to cell via gap junctions throughout the entire heart.*

The rate of spontaneous diastolic depolarization of the SA nodal cells (and thus the heart rate) is modulated by the autonomic nervous system.

 Excitation of the cardiac myocyte initiates contraction by increasing the cytosolic calcium level that activates the contractile apparatus.

 Mechanical response of the myocyte depends on preload (determined by the initial resting length), afterload (determined by the tension that needs to be developed), and contractility (the degree of activation of the contractile apparatus dependent on the amount of calcium released on activation).

 The cardiac myocyte length–tension relationships are correlated with changes in volume and pressure in the intact ventricle.

STUDY QUESTIONS

2–1. Small changes in extracellular potassium ion concentrations have major effects on cell membrane potentials.

    a. What will happen to the potassium equilibrium potential of cardiac muscle cells when interstitial $[K^+]$ (ie, $[K^+]_o$) is elevated?

    b. What effect will this have on the cells' resting membrane potential?

    c. What effect will this have on the cells' excitability?

2–2. Cardiac survival during cardiac transplantation is improved by perfusing donor hearts with cardioplegic solutions containing approximately 20 mM KCl. Why is this high potassium concentration helpful?

2–3. There are several classes of drugs that are useful for treating various cardiac arrhythmias. Identify the primary effects of each of the following classes of drugs on cardiac myocyte characteristics:

    a. What are the effects of sodium channel blockers on the PR interval of the ECG? On the duration of the QRS complex?

    b. What are the effects of calcium channel blockers on the rate of firing of SA nodal cells? On the rate of conduction of the action potential through the AV node? On myocardial contractility?

    c. What are the effects of potassium channel blockers on action potential duration? On refractory periods?

2–4. Very high sympathetic neural activity to the heart can lead to tetanic concentration of the cardiac muscle. True or false?

2–5. An increase in which of the following (with the others held constant) will result in an increase in the amount of active shortening of a cardiac muscle cell?

    a. preload

    b. afterload   shortening is less

    c. contractility

2–6. What happens when an intervention promotes early activation of the "delayed rectifier" K^+ channel (I_K) in a cardiac muscle?

 a. The resting potential is increased (hyperpolarized).
 b. The action potential duration is decreased.
 c. The action potential amplitude is decreased.
 d. The action potential conduction velocity is increased.
 e. The absolute refractory period is prolonged.

2–7. Action potential conduction velocity in cardiac muscle tissue is influenced by all of the following except

 a. cell diameter T
 b. resting membrane potential
 c. extracellular potassium concentration
 d. rate of rise (phase 0) of the action potential T
 e. duration of the plateau phase (phase 2) of the action potential T

2–8. The primary route of removal of $[Ca^{2+}]$ from the sarcoplasm during relaxation of a cardiac muscle cell is by

 a. active transport out of the cell
 b. passive exchange with extracellular sodium
 c. active transport into the sarcoplasmic reticulum
 d. trapping of calcium by troponin in the myofilaments
 e. passive movement out of the cell via L-type calcium channels

---

2-1   a.) the K⁺eq will be reduced, ↑ extracellular potassium will begin to abolish the driving force for K⁺ to leave the cell. The cell will begin to become depolarized. The cardiac myocyte looses it's ability to be excitable because hyperpolarization is essential to generate AP in cardiac myocytes.

2-2   ?

2-3 a.) Na⁺ blocker would prolong the PR interval and abolish the QRS complex

 b.) ↓ Rate of firing ↓Chronotropy; ↓ Conduction velocity ·dromotropy; ↓ myocardial contractility

 c.) a.p duration would persistand be really prolonged Repolarization would take a long time. It would extend Refractory periods

The Heart Pump

OBJECTIVES

The student knows the basic electrical and mechanical events of the cardiac cycle:
- ▶ *Correlates the electrocardiographic events with the mechanical events during the cardiac cycle.*
- ▶ *Lists the major distinct phases of the cardiac cycle as delineated by valve opening and closure.*
- ▶ *Describes the pressure and volume changes in the atria, the ventricles, and the aorta during each phase of the cardiac cycle.*
- ▶ *Defines and states normal values for (1) ventricular end-diastolic volume, end-systolic volume, stroke volume, diastolic pressure, and peak systolic pressure, and (2) aortic diastolic pressure, systolic pressure, and pulse pressure.*
- ▶ *States similarities and differences between mechanical events in the left and right heart pump.*
- ▶ *States the origin of the heart sounds.*
- ▶ *Diagrams the relationship between left ventricular pressure and volume during the cardiac cycle.*

The student understands the factors that determine cardiac output:
- ▶ *Defines cardiac output and cardiac index.*
- ▶ *States the relationship between cardiac output, the heart rate, and stroke volume.*
- ▶ *Identifies the major determinants of stroke volume.*
  - ▶ *States the Frank–Starling law of the heart.*
  - ▶ *Predicts the effect of altered ventricular preload on stroke volume and the ventricular pressure–volume relationship.*
  - ▶ *Predicts the effect of altered ventricular afterload on stroke volume and the ventricular pressure–volume relationship.*
  - ▶ *Predicts the effect of altered ventricular contractility (inotropic state) on stroke volume and the ventricular pressure–volume relationship.*
- ▶ *Draws a family of cardiac function curves describing the relationship between filling pressure and cardiac output under various levels of sympathetic tone.*
- ▶ *The student identifies the factors that influence myocardial oxygen consumption.*

The repetitive, synchronized contraction and relaxation of the cardiac muscle cells provide the forces necessary to pump blood through the systemic and pulmonary circulations. In this chapter, we describe (1) basic mechanical features of this cardiac pump, (2) factors that influence and/or regulate the cardiac output, and (3) sources of energy and energy costs required for myocardial activity.

CARDIAC CYCLE

Left Pump

The mechanical function of the heart can be described by the pressure, volume, and flow changes that occur within it during one cardiac cycle. A cardiac cycle is defined as one complete sequence of contraction and relaxation. The normal mechanical events of a cycle of the left heart pump are correlated in Figure 3–1. This important figure summarizes a great deal of information and should be studied carefully.

VENTRICULAR DIASTOLE

The *diastolic phase*[1] of the cardiac cycle begins with the opening of the atrioventricular (AV) valves. As shown in Figure 3–1, the mitral valve opens when left ventricular pressure falls below left atrial pressure and the period of ventricle filling begins. Blood that had previously accumulated in the atrium behind the closed mitral valve empties rapidly into the ventricle, and this causes an initial drop in atrial pressure. Later, the pressures in both chambers slowly rise together as the atrium and ventricle continue passively filling in unison with blood returning to the heart through the veins.

Atrial contraction is initiated near the end of ventricular diastole by the depolarization of the atrial muscle cells, which causes the P wave of the electrocardiogram. As the atrial muscle cells develop tension and shorten, atrial pressure rises and an additional amount of blood is forced into the ventricle. At normal heart rates, atrial contraction is not essential for adequate ventricular filling. This is evident in Figure 3–1 from the fact that the ventricle has nearly reached its maximum or *end-diastolic volume* before atrial contraction begins. Atrial contraction plays an increasingly significant role in ventricular filling as heart rate increases because the time interval between beats for passive filling becomes progressively shorter with increased heart rate. Note that throughout diastole, atrial and ventricular pressures are nearly identical. This is because a normal open mitral valve has very little resistance to flow and thus only a very small atrial–ventricular pressure difference is necessary to produce ventricular filling.

VENTRICULAR SYSTOLE

Ventricular systole begins when the action potential breaks through the AV node and sweeps over the ventricular muscle—an event heralded by the QRS complex of the electrocardiogram. Contraction of the ventricular muscle cells causes intraventricular pressure to rise above that in the atrium, which causes abrupt closure of the AV valve. LUB Heart Sound

Pressure in the left ventricle continues to rise sharply as the ventricular contraction intensifies. When the left ventricular pressure exceeds that in the aorta, the aortic valve opens. The period between mitral valve closure and aortic valve opening is referred to as the *isovolumetric contraction phase* because during this interval the

---

[1] The atria and ventricles do not beat simultaneously. Usually, and unless otherwise noted, systole and diastole denote phases of ventricular operation.

Figure 3–1. Cardiac cycle—left heart pump. Cardiac cycle phases: **A**, diastole; **B**, systole that is divided into three periods; **C**, isovolumetric contraction; **D**, ejection; and **E**, isovolumetric relaxation.

ventricle is a closed chamber with a fixed volume. Ventricular ejection begins with the opening of the aortic valve. In early ejection, blood enters the aorta rapidly and causes the pressure there to rise. Pressure builds simultaneously in both the ventricle and the aorta as the ventricular muscle cells continue to contract in early systole. This interval is often called the *rapid ejection period*.

Left ventricular and aortic pressures ultimately reach a maximum called *peak systolic pressure*. At this point the strength of ventricular muscle contraction begins to wane. Muscle shortening and ejection continue, but at a reduced rate. Aortic pressure begins to fall because blood is leaving the aorta and large arteries faster than blood is entering from the left ventricle. Throughout ejection, very small pressure differences exist between the left ventricle and the aorta because the aortic valve orifice is so large that it presents very little resistance to flow.

Eventually, the strength of the ventricular contraction diminishes to the point where intraventricular pressure falls below aortic pressure. This causes abrupt closure of the aortic valve. A dip, called the *incisura* or *dicrotic notch*, appears in the aortic pressure trace because a small volume of aortic blood must flow backward to fill the space behind the aortic valve leaflets as they close. After aortic valve closure, intraventricular pressure falls rapidly as the ventricular muscle relaxes. For a brief interval, called the *isovolumetric relaxation phase*, the mitral valve is also closed. Ultimately, intraventricular pressure falls below atrial pressure, the AV valve opens, and a new cardiac cycle begins.

Note that atrial pressure progressively rises during ventricular systole because blood continues to return to the heart and fill the atrium. The elevated atrial pressure at the end of systole promotes rapid ventricular filling once the AV valve opens to begin the next heart cycle.

The ventricle has reached its minimum or *end-systolic volume* at the time of aortic valve closure. The amount of blood ejected from the ventricle during a single beat, the *stroke volume*, is equal to ventricular end-diastolic volume minus ventricular end-systolic volume. $SV = EDV - ESV$

The aorta distends or balloons out during systole because more blood enters the aorta than leaves it. During diastole, the arterial pressure is maintained by the elastic recoil of walls of the aorta and other large arteries. Nonetheless, aortic pressure gradually falls during diastole as the aorta supplies blood to the systemic vascular beds. The lowest aortic pressure, reached at the end of diastole, is called *diastolic pressure*. The difference between diastolic and peak systolic pressures in the aorta is called the arterial *pulse pressure*. Typical values for systolic and diastolic pressures in the aorta are 120 and 80 mmHg, respectively.

At a normal resting heart rate of about 70 beats per minute, the heart spends approximately two-thirds of the cardiac cycle in diastole and one-third in systole. When increases in the heart rate occur, both diastolic and systolic intervals become shorter. Action potential durations are shortened and conduction velocity is increased. Contraction and relaxation rates are also enhanced. This shortening of the systolic interval tends to blunt the potential adverse effects of increases in the heart rate on diastolic filling time.

Right Pump

Because the entire heart is served by a single electrical excitation system, similar mechanical events occur essentially simultaneously in both the left and right sides of the heart. Both ventricles have synchronous systolic and

24/8 Kobe

25/8 mmHg

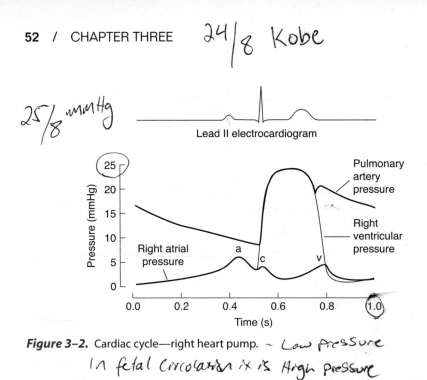

Lead II electrocardiogram

Figure 3–2. Cardiac cycle—right heart pump. ~ Low Pressure

In fetal Circulation it is High pressure

diastolic periods, and the valves of the right and left sides of the heart normally open and close nearly in unison. Because the two sides of the heart are arranged in series in the circulation, they must pump the same amount of blood and therefore must have identical stroke volumes.

The major difference between the right and left pumps is in the magnitude of the peak systolic pressure. The pressures developed by the right side of the heart as shown in Figure 3–2 are considerably lower than those for the left side of the heart (Figure 3–1). This is because the lungs provide considerably less resistance to blood flow than that offered collectively by the systemic organs. Therefore, less arterial pressure is required to drive the cardiac output through the lungs than through the systemic organs. Typical pulmonary artery systolic and diastolic pressures are 24 and 8 mmHg, respectively.

The pressure pulsations that occur in the right atrium are transmitted in retrograde fashion to the large veins near the heart. These pulsations, shown on the atrial pressure trace in Figure 3–2, can be visualized in the neck over the jugular veins in a recumbent individual. They are collectively referred to as the *jugular venous pulse* and can provide clinically useful information about the heart. Atrial contraction produces the first pressure peak called the *a* wave. The *c* wave, which follows shortly thereafter, coincides with the onset of ventricular systole and is caused by an initial bulging of the tricuspid valve into the right atrium. Right atrial pressure falls after the *c* wave because of atrial relaxation and a downward displacement of the tricuspid valve during ventricular emptying. Right atrial pressure then begins to increase toward a third peak, the *v* wave, as the central veins and right atrium fill behind a closed tricuspid valve with blood returning to the heart from the peripheral organs. With the opening of the tricuspid valve at the conclusion of ventricular systole, right atrial pressure again falls as blood moves into the relaxed right ventricle.

Shortly afterward, right atrial pressure begins to rise once more toward the next *a* wave as returning blood fills the central veins, the right atrium, and right ventricle together during diastole.

Heart Sounds

A phonocardiographic record of the heart sounds, which occur in the cardiac cycle, is included in Figure 3–1. These sounds are normally heard by *auscultation* with a stethoscope placed on the chest. The first heart sound, S_1, occurs at the beginning of systole because of the abrupt closure of the AV valves, which produces vibrations of the cardiac structures and the blood in the ventricular chambers. S_1 can be heard most clearly by placing the stethoscope over the apex of the heart. Note that this sound occurs immediately after the QRS complex of the electrocardiogram.

The second heart sound, S_2, arises from the closure of the aortic and pulmonic valves at the beginning of the period of isovolumetric relaxation. This sound is heard at near the end of the T wave in the electrocardiogram. The pulmonic valve usually closes slightly after the aortic valve. Because this discrepancy is enhanced during the inspiratory phase of the respiratory cycle, inspiration causes what is referred to as the *physiological splitting of the second heart sound*. The discrepancy in valve closure during inspiration may range from 30 to 60 ms. One of the factors that lead to prolonged ejection of the right ventricle during inspiration is that the decreased intrathoracic pressure that accompanies inspiration transiently enhances venous return and diastolic filling of the right side of the heart. For reasons that are detailed later in this chapter, this extra filling volume will be ejected but a little extra time is required to do so.

The third and fourth heart sounds, shown in Figure 3–1, are not normally present. When they are present, however, they, along with S_1 and S_2, produce what are called *gallop rhythms* (resembling the sound of a galloping horse). When present, the third heart sound occurs shortly after S_2 during the period of rapid passive ventricular filling and, in combination with heart sounds S_1 and S_2, produces what is called *ventricular gallop rhythm*. Although S_3 may sometimes be detected in normal children, it is heard more commonly in patients with left ventricular failure. The fourth heart sound, which occasionally is heard shortly before S_1, is associated with atrial contraction and rapid active filling of the ventricle. Thus, the combination of S_1, S_2, and S_4 sounds produces what is called an *atrial gallop rhythm*. The presence of S_4 often indicates an increased ventricular diastolic stiffness, which can occur with several cardiac disease states.

Cardiac Cycle Pressure–Volume and Length–Tension Relationships

Intraventricular pressure and volume are intimately linked to the tension and length of the cardiac muscle cells in the ventricular wall through purely geometric and physical laws. Figures 3–3A and 3–3B show the correspondence between a ventricular pressure–volume loop and a cardiac muscle length–tension

Handwritten annotations:
aortic valve closes @ Higher pressure than it opened
S2
aortic valve closes
Sys tole
1 cardiac cycle
ESV
afterload! pressure required to open Aortic valve
EDV
Mitral valve closes
S1 preload

A

Intraventricular pressure (mmHg)

120

80

Reaches end-systolic volume

Ejection

Aortic valve opens

Systole

Isovolumetric relaxation

Isovolumetric contraction

Mitral valve opens

Diastolic filling

Reaches end-diastolic volume

60

130

Stroke volume
Intraventricular volume (mL)

B

Muscle tension

Shortening

Reaches end-systolic length

Active

Isometric tension development

Isometric relaxation

Passive stretch

Reaches end-diastolic length

Muscle length

Figure 3–3. (**A**) Left ventricular pressure–volume cycle and (**B**) corresponding cardiac muscle length–tension cycle.

loop during one cardiac cycle. This fact makes it clear that cardiac muscle length–tension behavior is the underlying basis for ventricular function. Note that in Figure 3–3, each major phase of the ventricular cardiac cycle has a corresponding phase of cardiac muscle length and tension change. During diastolic ventricular filling, for example, the progressive increase in ventricular pressure causes a corresponding increase in muscle tension, which passively stretches the resting cardiac muscle to greater lengths along its resting length–tension curve. End-diastolic ventricular pressure is referred to as *ventricular preload* because it sets the end-diastolic ventricular

Example:
aortic stenosis — ↑ in afterload ↓ in Shortening ↓ SV ● ↑ IV pressure required
aortic Regurg. — ↑ in preload ↑ EDV ↑ Resting length tension ↑ SV
CHF
CKD
Edema

volume and therefore the resting length of the cardiac muscle fibers at the end of diastole.

At the onset of systole, the ventricular muscle cells develop tension isometrically and intraventricular pressure rises accordingly. After the intraventricular pressure rises sufficiently to open the outlet valve, ventricular ejection begins as a consequence of ventricular muscle shortening. Systemic arterial pressure is often referred to as the *ventricular afterload* because it determines the tension that must be developed by cardiac muscle fibers before they can shorten.[2]

During cardiac ejection, the cardiac muscle is simultaneously generating active tension *and* shortening (ie, an afterloaded isotonic contraction). The magnitude of ventricular volume change during ejection (ie, stroke volume) is determined simply by how far ventricular muscle cells are able to shorten during contraction. This, as already discussed, depends on the length–tension relationship of the cardiac muscle cells and the load against which they are shortening. Once shortening ceases and the output valve closes, the cardiac muscle cells relax isometrically. Ventricular wall tension and intraventricular pressure fall in unison during isovolumetric relaxation.

DETERMINANTS OF CARDIAC OUTPUT

Cardiac output (liters of blood pumped by *each* of the ventricles per minute) is an extremely important cardiovascular variable that is continuously adjusted so that the cardiovascular system operates to meet the body's moment-to-moment transport needs. In going from rest to strenuous exercise, for example, the cardiac output of an average person will increase from approximately 5.5 to perhaps 15 L/min. The extra cardiac output provides the exercising skeletal muscles with the additional nutritional supply needed to sustain an increased metabolic rate. To understand the cardiovascular system's response not only to exercise but to all other physiological or pathological demands placed on it, we must understand what determines and therefore controls cardiac output.

As stated in Chapter 1, cardiac output is the product of the heart rate and stroke volume (CO = HR × SV). Therefore, all changes in cardiac output must be produced by changes in the heart rate and/or stroke volume. − EDV & ESV

Factors influencing the heart rate do so by altering the characteristics of the diastolic depolarization of the pacemaker cells as discussed in Chapter 2 (Figure 2–6). Recall that variations in activity of the sympathetic and parasympathetic nerves leading to cells of the sinoatrial (SA) node constitute the most important regulators of the heart rate. Increases in sympathetic activity increase the heart rate, whereas increases in parasympathetic activity decrease the heart rate. These neural inputs have

---

[2] This designation is somewhat misleading for at least two reasons. First, arterial pressure is more analogous to ventricular total load than to ventricular afterload. Second, because of the law of Laplace, the actual wall tension that needs to be generated to attain a given intraventricular pressure also depends on the ventricular radius (tension = pressure × radius). Thus, the larger the end-diastolic volume, the greater the tension required to develop sufficient intraventricular pressure to open the outflow valve. We choose, however, to ignore these complications at this time.

immediate effects (within one beat) and therefore can cause very rapid adjustments in cardiac output.

INFLUENCES ON STROKE VOLUME

Effect of Changes in Ventricular Preload: Frank–Starling Law of the Heart

The volume of blood that the heart ejects with each beat can vary significantly. One of the most important factors responsible for these variations in stroke volume is the extent of cardiac filling during diastole. This concept is introduced in Chapter 1 (Figure 1–7) and is known as Starling's law of the heart. To review (and to reemphasize its importance), this law states that, with other factors equal, *stroke volume increases as cardiac filling increases*. As shown below, this phenomenon is based on the intrinsic mechanical properties of myocardial muscle.

Figure 3–4A illustrates how increasing muscle preload will increase the extent of shortening during a subsequent contraction with a fixed total load. Recall from

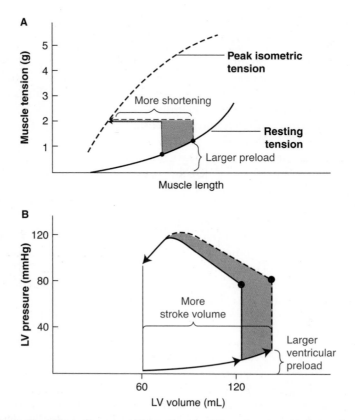

Figure 3–4. The effect of increased in preload on (**A**) cardiac muscle shortening during afterloaded contractions and (**B**) ventricular stroke volume.

the nature of the resting length–tension relationship that an increased preload is necessarily accompanied by increased initial muscle fiber length. As described in Chapter 2, when a muscle starts from a greater length, it has more distance to shorten before it reaches the length at which its tension-generating capability is no longer greater than the load on it. The same behavior is exhibited by cardiac muscle cells when they are actually operating in the ventricular wall. Increases in ventricular preload increase both end-diastolic volume and stroke volume almost equally, as illustrated in Figure 3–4B.

The precise relationship between cardiac preload (cardiac filling pressure) and end-diastolic volume has especially important physiological and clinical consequences. Although the actual relationship is somewhat curvilinear, especially at very high filling pressures, it is nearly linear over the normal operating range of the heart. The low slope of this relationship indicates the incredible distensibility of the normal ventricle during diastole (eg, a change in filling pressure of only 1 mmHg normally will change end-diastolic volume by about 25 mL). As discussed in Chapter 11, one major form of cardiac failure is called "diastolic failure" and is characterized by a decidedly abnormal relationship between cardiac filling pressure and end-diastolic volume.

It should be noted in Figure 3–4A that increasing preload increases initial muscle length without significantly changing the final length to which the muscle shortens against a constant total load. Thus, increasing ventricular filling pressure increases stroke volume primarily by increasing end-diastolic volume. As shown in Figure 3–4B, this is not accompanied by a significant alteration in end-systolic volume.

Effect of Changes in Ventricular Afterload

As stated previously, systemic arterial pressure is usually taken to be the left ventricular "afterload". A slight complication is that arterial pressure varies between a diastolic value and a systolic value during each cardiac ejection. Usually, however, we are interested in *mean* ventricular afterload and take this to be *mean* arterial pressure.

Figure 3–5A shows how increased afterload, at constant preload, has a negative effect on cardiac muscle shortening. Again, this is simply a consequence of the fact that muscle cannot shorten beyond the length at which its peak isometric tension-generating potential equals the total load on it. Thus, shortening must stop at a greater muscle length when afterload is increased.

Normally, mean ventricular afterload is quite constant, because mean arterial pressure is held within tight limits by the cardiovascular control mechanisms described later. In many pathological situations such as hypertension and aortic valve obstruction, however, ventricular function is adversely influenced by abnormally high ventricular afterload. When this occurs, stroke volume may be decreased as shown by the changes in the pressure–volume loop in Figure 3–5B. Under these conditions, note that stroke volume is decreased because end-systolic volume is increased.

The relationship between end-systolic pressure and end-systolic volume obtained at a constant preload but different afterloads is indicated by the dotted

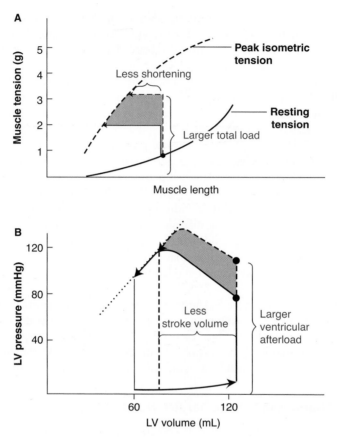

Figure 3–5. The effect of increased in afterload on (**A**) cardiac muscle shortening during afterloaded contractions and (**B**) ventricular stroke volume.

line in Figure 3–5B. In a normally functioning heart, the effect of changes in afterload on end-systolic volume (and therefore stroke volume) is quite small (about 0.5 mL/mmHg). However, in what is termed "systolic cardiac failure," the effect of afterload on end-systolic volume is greatly enhanced. Thus, the slope of this line can be used clinically to assess the systolic function of the heart as discussed further in Chapter 11.

Effect of Changes in Cardiac Muscle Contractility

Recall that activation of the sympathetic nervous system results in release of norepinephrine from cardiac sympathetic nerves, which increases contractility of the individual cardiac muscle cells. This results in an upward shift of the peak isometric length–tension curve. As shown in Figure 3–6A, such a shift will result in an increase in the shortening of a muscle contracting with constant preload and total load. Thus, as shown in Figure 3–6B, the norepinephrine released by sympathetic nerve stimulation will increase ventricular stroke volume by decreasing the end-systolic volume, without directly influencing the end-diastolic volume.

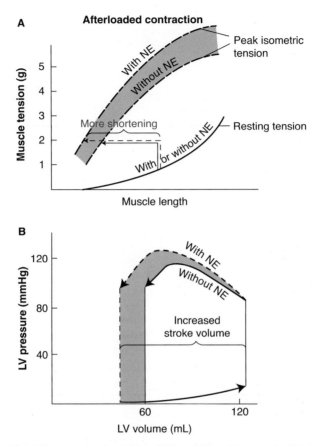

Figure 3–6. The effect of norepinephrine (NE) on (**A**) cardiac muscle shortening during afterloaded contractions and (**B**) ventricular stroke volume.

In addition to this change in the extent of myocyte shortening, an increase in contractility will also cause an increase in the *rates* of myocyte tension development and of shortening. This will result in an increase in the *rate* of isovolumetric pressure development and the *rate* of ejection during systole.

SUMMARY OF DETERMINANTS OF CARDIAC OUTPUT

The major influences on cardiac output are summarized in Figure 3–7. The heart rate is controlled by chronotropic influences on the spontaneous electrical activity of SA nodal cells. Cardiac parasympathetic nerves have a negative chronotropic effect, and sympathetic nerves have a positive chronotropic effect on the SA node. Stroke volume is controlled by influences on the contractile performance of the ventricular cardiac muscle—in particular, its degree of shortening in the afterloaded situation. The three distinct influences on stroke volume are contractility, preload, and afterload. Increased cardiac sympathetic nerve activity tends to increase stroke

Figure 3–7. Influences on cardiac output.

volume by increasing the contractility of the cardiac muscle. Increased arterial pressure tends to decrease stroke volume by increasing the afterload on cardiac muscle fibers. Increased ventricular filling pressure increases end-diastolic volume, which tends to increase stroke volume through Starling's law.

It is important to recognize at this point that both the heart rate and stroke volume are subject to more than one influence. Thus, the fact that increased contractility tends to increase stroke volume should not be taken to mean that, in the intact cardiovascular system, stroke volume is always high when contractility is high. Following blood loss caused by hemorrhage, for example, stroke volume may be low in spite of a high level of sympathetic nerve activity and increased contractility. The only other possible causes for low stroke volume are high arterial pressure and low cardiac filling pressure. Because arterial pressure is normal or low following hemorrhage, the low stroke volume associated with severe blood loss must be (and is) the result of low cardiac filling pressure.

Cardiac Function Curves

One very useful way to summarize the influences on cardiac function and the interactions between them is by cardiac function curves such as those shown in Figure 3–8.

 In this case, cardiac output is treated as the dependent variable and is plotted on the vertical axis in Figure 3–8, while cardiac filling pressure is plotted on the horizontal axis.[3]

---

[3] Other variables may appear on the axes of these curves. The vertical axis may be designated as stroke volume or stroke work, whereas the horizontal axis may be designated as central venous pressure, right (or left) atrial

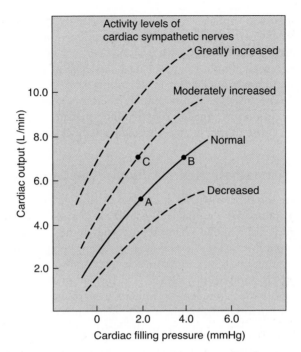

Figure 3–8. Influence of cardiac sympathetic nerves on cardiac function curves.

Different curves are used to show the influence of alterations in cardiac sympathetic nerve activity. Thus, Figure 3–8 shows how the cardiac filling pressure and the activity level of cardiac sympathetic nerves interact to determine cardiac output. When cardiac filling pressure is 2 mmHg and the activity of cardiac sympathetic nerves is normal, the heart will operate at point A and will have a cardiac output of 5 L/min. Each single curve in Figure 3–8 shows how cardiac output would be changed by changes in cardiac filling pressure if cardiac sympathetic nerve activity were held at a fixed level. For example, if cardiac sympathetic nerve activity remained normal, increasing cardiac filling pressure from 2 to 4 mmHg would cause the heart to shift its operation from point A to point B on the cardiac function diagram. In this case, cardiac output would increase from 5 to 7 L/min solely as a result of the increased filling pressure (Starling's law). If, on the other hand, cardiac filling pressure were fixed at 2 mmHg while the activity of cardiac sympathetic nerves was moderately increased from normal, the heart would change from operating at point A to operating at point C. Cardiac output would again increase from 5 to 7 L/min. In this instance, however, cardiac output does not increase through the length-dependent mechanism because cardiac filling pressure did not change. Cardiac output increases at constant filling pressure with an increase in cardiac sympathetic activity for two

pressure, or ventricular end-diastolic volume (or pressure). In all cases, the curves describe the relationship between preload and cardiac function.

reasons. First, increased cardiac sympathetic nerve activity increases the heart rate. Second, but just as importantly, increased sympathetic nerve activity increases stroke volume by increasing cardiac contractility.[4]

Cardiac function graphs thus consolidate knowledge of many mechanisms of cardiac control and are most helpful in describing how the heart interacts with other elements in the cardiovascular system. Furthermore, these graphs reemphasize the important point that a change in cardiac filling pressure alone will have a very potent effect on cardiac output at any level of sympathetic activity.

Summary of Sympathetic Neural Influences on Cardiac Function

Because of its importance in overall control of cardiac function, it is appropriate at this point to summarize the major direct effects that the sympathetic nervous system exerts on electrical and mechanical properties of the cardiac muscle and thus on cardiac pumping ability. These effects are initiated by norepinephrine interaction with β_1-adrenergic receptors on cardiac muscle cells, resulting in a cascade of events involving the G_s activation of adenylate cyclase, formation of cAMP, and activation of protein kinase A with subsequent phosphorylation of many molecules that play key regulatory roles in intracellular processes. These cellular events combine to evoke improvements in pumping capabilities of the heart. These improvements include the following:

1. An increase in the heart rate (positive chronotropic effect) by activating the inward-going sodium i_f current in SA nodal cells;

2. A decrease in cardiac action potential duration by early activation of the delayed i_K current in cardiac myocytes, which minimizes the detrimental effect of high heart rates on diastolic filling time;

3. An increase in the rate of action potential conduction, particularly evident in the AV node (positive dromotropic effect) by altering conductivity of gap junctions;

4. An increase in cardiac contractility (positive inotropic effect) by activating the $i_{Ca^{2+}}$ current and increasing Ca^{2+} release from the sarcoplasmic reticulum, which increases the contractile ability of the cardiac muscle at any given preload; and

5. An increase in the rate of cardiac relaxation (positive lusitropic effect) by increasing Ca^{2+} uptake by the sarcoplasmic reticulum, which also helps minimize the detrimental effect of high heart rates on diastolic filling time.[5,6]

---

[4] Decreases in cardiac afterload can also shift the position of the curve upward by allowing more shortening to occur at a given preload. This effect is normally not important because afterload is usually kept constant.
[5] Most catecholamine effects on the heart are a result of increases in sympathetic neural activity. Although circulating catecholamines of adrenal origin can potentially evoke similar effects, their concentrations are normally so low that their contributions are negligible.
[6] All the effects of catecholamines on cardiac muscle can be blocked by specific drugs called β-adrenergic receptor blockers. The drugs may be useful in the treatment of coronary artery disease to thwart increased metabolic demands placed on the heart by activity of sympathetic nerves.

As shown in subsequent chapters, increases in sympathetic activity can have *indirect* influences on cardiac function that are a consequence of sympathetic-induced alterations in arteriolar and venous tone (ie, alterations in afterload and preload, respectively).

CARDIAC ENERGETICS

Energy Sources

In order for the heart to operate properly, it must have an adequate supply of chemical energy in the form of adenosine triphosphate (ATP). The relatively low ATP content of cardiac tissue combined with a relatively high rate of ATP hydrolysis at rest suggests that the myocardial ATP pool will completely turn over every 10 seconds.

The substrates from which ATP is formed by the heart depend partly on which substrates are in the greatest supply at a particular instant. For example, after a high-carbohydrate meal, the heart will take up and metabolize glucose and pyruvate, whereas between meals, the heart can switch to metabolize free fatty acids, triglycerides, and ketones. Unlike the skeletal muscle, the cardiac muscle can utilize lactate as an energy source, which is beneficial during strenuous exercise when skeletal muscles are producing lactate. In addition, the choice of substrate depends on the metabolic phenotype of the cardiac muscle. Fetal and newborn hearts derive most of their ATP from metabolism of glucose and lactate, whereas, within a few weeks of birth, a switch toward fatty acid oxidation occurs so that, by adulthood, 60 to 90% of cardiac ATP is derived from fatty acids. A switch back toward the fetal phenotype accompanies severe heart failure. Glycogen is stored in myocardial cells as a reserve energy supply and can be mobilized via the glycolytic pathway to provide extra substrate under conditions of increased sympathetic stimulation.

The end product of metabolism of glycogen, glucose, fatty acids, triglycerides, pyruvate, and lactate is acetyl CoA, which enters the citric acid (Krebs) cycle in the mitochondria, where, by a process of oxidative phosphorylation, the molecules are degraded to carbon dioxide and water and the energy is converted to ATP. (The student is encouraged to consult a biochemistry textbook for further details of these important metabolic pathways.)

The anaerobic sources of energy in the heart (eg, glycolysis and creatine phosphate) are not adequate to sustain the metabolic demand for more than a few minutes. The heavy (nearly total) reliance of the heart on the aerobic pathways for ATP production is evident by (1) the high number of mitochondria and (2) the presence of high concentrations of the oxygen-binding protein myoglobin within the cardiac muscle cells. Myoglobin can release its oxygen to the mitochondrial cytochrome oxidase system when intracellular oxygen levels are lowered. In these regards, the cardiac muscle resembles "red" skeletal muscle that is adapted for sustained contractile activity as opposed to "white" skeletal muscle that is adapted for high-intensity, short-duration contractile activity.

Determinants of Myocardial Oxygen Consumption

In many pathological situations, such as obstructive coronary artery disease, the oxygen requirements of the myocardial tissue may exceed the capacity of coronary blood flow to deliver oxygen to the heart muscle. It is important to understand what factors determine the energy costs and, therefore, the myocardial oxygen consumption rate because reduction of the oxygen demand may be of significant clinical benefit to the patient.

Because the heart derives its energy almost entirely from aerobic metabolism, myocardial oxygen consumption is directly related to myocardial energy use (ie, ATP splitting). Understanding the determinants of myocardial oxygen consumption essentially means understanding the myocardial processes that require ATP.

The *basal metabolism* of the heart tissue normally accounts for about 25% of myocardial ATP use and therefore myocardial oxygen consumption in a resting individual. Because basal metabolism represents the energy consumed in cellular processes other than contraction (eg, energy-dependent ion pumping), little can be done to reduce it.

The processes associated with *muscle contraction* account for about 75% of myocardial energy use. Primarily, this reflects ATP splitting associated with cross-bridge cycling during the isovolumetric contraction and ejection phases of the cardiac cycle. Some ATP is also used for Ca^{2+} sequestration at the termination of each contraction.

The energy expended during the isovolumetric contraction phase of the cardiac cycle accounts for the largest portion ($\sim$50%) of total myocardial oxygen consumption despite the fact that the heart does no external work during this period. The energy needed for isovolumetric contraction depends heavily on the intraventricular pressure that must develop during this time, that is, on the cardiac afterload. *Cardiac afterload* then is a major determinant of myocardial oxygen consumption. Reductions in cardiac afterload can produce clinically significant reductions in myocardial energy requirements and therefore myocardial oxygen consumption.

Energy utilization during isovolumetric contraction is actually more directly related to isometric *wall tension* development than to intraventricular pressure development. Recall that wall tension is related to intraventricular pressure *and* ventricular radius through the law of Laplace ($T = P \times r$). Consequently, reductions in cardiac preload (ie, end-diastolic volume and radius) will also tend to reduce the energy required for isovolumetric contraction.

It is during the ejection phase of the cardiac cycle when the heart actually performs external work and the energy the heart expends during ejection depends on how much *external work* it is doing. In a fluid system, work (force × distance) is equal to pressure (force/distance^2) × volume (distance^3). The external physical work done by the left ventricle in one beat, called *stroke work*, is equal to the area enclosed by the left ventricular pressure–volume loop (see Figure 3–3). Stroke work is increased either by an increase in stroke volume (increased "volume" work) or by an increase in afterload (increased "pressure" work). In terms of ATP utilization and oxygen consumption, increases in the pressure work of the heart are more costly than increases in volume work. Thus, reductions in afterload are especially helpful in reducing the myocardial oxygen requirements for doing external work.

Changes in *myocardial contractility* can have important consequences on the oxygen requirement for basal metabolism, isovolumic wall tension generation, and external work. Heart muscle cells use more energy in rapidly developing a given tension and shortening by a given amount than in doing the same thing more slowly. Also, with increased contractility, more energy is expended in active Ca^{2+} transport. The net result of these influences is often referred to as the "energy wasting" effect of increased contractility.

The *heart rate* is one of the most important determinants of myocardial oxygen consumption because the energy costs per minute must equal the energy cost per beat times the number of beats per minute. In general, it has been found that it is more efficient (less oxygen is required) to achieve a given cardiac output with the low heart rate and high stroke volume than with the high heart rate and low stroke volume. This again appears to be related to the relatively high energy cost of the pressure development phase of the cardiac cycle. The less pressure (wall tension) developed and the less often pressure development occurs, the better.

KEY CONCEPTS

(1) *Effective cardiac pumping of blood requires coordinated filling of the chambers, excitation and contraction of the cardiac muscle cells, pressure generation within the chambers, opening and closing of cardiac valves, and one-way movement of blood through the chambers into the aorta or pulmonary artery.*

(2) *Except for lower ejection pressures, events of the right side of the heart are identical to those of the left side.*

(3) *Heart sounds associated with valve movements and detected on auscultation can be used to identify the beginnings of diastolic and systolic phases of the cardiac cycle.*

(4) *The events of a single ventricular cardiac cycle can be displayed as records of electrical, mechanical, pressure, sound or flow changes against time or as a record of volume against pressure.*

(5) *Cardiac output is defined as the amount of blood pumped by either of the ventricles per minute and is determined by the product of the heart rate and stroke volume.*

(6) *Stroke volume can be altered by changes in ventricular preload (filling), ventricular afterload (arterial pressure), and/or cardiac muscle contractility.*

(7) *A cardiac function curve describes the relationship between ventricular filling and cardiac output and can be shifted up (left) or down (right) by changes in sympathetic activity to the heart or by changes in cardiac muscle contractility.*

(8) *Energy for cardiac muscle contraction is derived primarily from aerobic metabolic pathways such that cardiac work is tightly related to myocardial oxygen consumption.*

STUDY QUESTIONS

3–1. If pulmonary artery pressure is 24/8 mmHg (systolic/diastolic), what are the respective systolic and diastolic pressures of the right ventricle? *24/8*

3–2. Because pulmonary artery pressure is so much lower than aortic pressure, the right ventricle has a larger stroke volume than the left ventricle. True or *false?*

3–3. Which of the following interventions will increase cardiac stroke volume?
  a. increased ventricular filling pressure
  b. decreased arterial pressure
  c. increased activity of cardiac sympathetic nerves
  ~~d.~~ increased circulating catecholamine levels

3–4. In which direction will cardiac output change if central venous pressure is lowered while cardiac sympathetic tone is increased? *— no not change*

3–5. Increases in sympathetic neural activity to the heart will result in an increase in stroke volume by causing a decrease in end-systolic volume for any given end-diastolic volume. *True* or false?

3–6. Four of these conditions exist during the same phase of the cardiac cycle and one does not. Which one is the odd one?
  a. The mitral valve is open.
  b. The QRS wave of the ECG is occurring.
  c. The "v" wave of the jugular venous pulse has just occurred.
  d. Ventricular volume is rapidly increasing.
  e. Aortic pressure is falling.

3–7. With all other factors equal, myocardial oxygen demands will be increased to the greatest extent by which of the following?
  a. increases in the heart rate
  b. increases in coronary flow
  c. increases in end-diastolic volume
  d. decreases in arterial pressure
  e. decreases in cardiac contractility

3–8. Sympathetic neural activation of the heart will decrease which of the following?
  a. ~~heart rate~~
  b. PR interval on the ECG
  c. metabolic demands
  d. coronary flow rate
  e. ~~cardiac contractility~~

Measurements of Cardiac Function

4

OBJECTIVES

The student recognizes several techniques of assessing cardiac output and cardiac contractility:

▶ *Given data, calculates cardiac output using the Fick principle.*

▶ *Defines ejection fraction and identifies visualization methods used to determine it.*

▶ *Describes the end-systolic pressure–volume relationship.*

The student understands the physiological basis of the electrocardiogram:

▶ *States the relationship between electrical events of cardiac excitation and the P, QRS, and T waves, the PR and QT intervals, and the ST segment of the electrocardiogram.*

▶ *States Einthoven's basic electrocardiographic conventions and, given data, determines the mean electrical axis of the heart.*

▶ *Describes the standard 12-lead electrocardiogram.*

There are a variety of methods available to assess cardiac function. Some of these are noninvasive (eg, auscultation of the chest to evaluate valve function, electrocardiography to evaluate electrical characteristics, and echocardiography to visualize mechanical pumping action) and others require various types of invasive instrumentation. This chapter provides a brief overview of some of these commonly used clinical tools.

MEASUREMENT OF CARDIAC OUTPUT

Fick principle is one of the most accurate methods of measuring cardiac output, which is discussed in detail in Chapter 6. Briefly, this principle states that the amount of a substance consumed by the tissues, X_{tc}, is equal to what goes in minus what goes out, which is the arterial–venous concentration difference in the substance ($[X]_a - [X]_v$) times the blood flow rate, $\dot{Q}$. This relationship can be algebraically arranged to solve for blood flow:

$$\dot{Q} = \frac{\dot{X}_{tc}}{[X]_a - [X]_v}$$

A common method of determining cardiac output is to use the Fick principle to calculate the collective flow through the systemic organs from (1) the whole body oxygen consumption rate ($\dot{X}_{tc}$), (2) the oxygen concentration in arterial blood ($[X]_a$), and (3) the concentration of oxygen in mixed venous blood ($[X]_v$). Of the values required for this calculation, the oxygen content of mixed venous blood is the most difficult to obtain. Generally, the sample for venous blood oxygen measurement must be taken from venous catheters positioned in the right ventricle or pulmonary artery to ensure that it is a mixed sample of venous blood from all systemic organs.

The calculation of cardiac output from the Fick principle is best illustrated by an example. Suppose that a patient is consuming 250 mL of O_2 per minute when his or her systemic arterial blood contains 200 mL of O_2 per liter and the right ventricular blood contains 150 mL of O_2 per liter. This means that, on the average, each liter of blood loses 50 mL of O_2 as it passes through the systemic organs. In order for 250 mL of O_2 to be consumed per minute, 5 L of blood must pass through the systemic circulation each minute:

$$\dot{Q} = \frac{250 \text{ mL } O_2/\text{min}}{200 - 150 \text{ mL } O_2/\text{L blood}}$$

$$\dot{Q} = 5 \text{ L blood/min}$$

Dye dilution and *thermal dilution* (dilution of heat) are other clinical techniques employed for estimating cardiac output. Usually, a known quantity of indicator (dye or heat) is rapidly injected into the blood as it enters the right side of the heart and appropriate detectors are arranged to continuously record the concentration of the indicator in blood as it leaves the left side of the heart. It is possible to estimate the cardiac output from the quantity of indicator injected and the time record of indicator concentration in the blood that leaves the left side of the heart.

Cardiac index is the cardiac output corrected for the individual's size. For example, the cardiac output of a 50-kg woman will be significantly lower than that of a 90-kg man. It has been found, however, that cardiac output correlates better with body surface area than with body weight. Therefore, it is common to express the cardiac output per square meter of surface area. Under resting conditions, the cardiac index is normally approximately 3 L/min per m^2.

CARDIAC CONTRACTILITY ESTIMATES

Imaging Techniques

 It is often important to assess an individual's cardiac function without using major invasive procedures. Advances in several techniques have made it possible to obtain two- and three-dimensional images of the heart throughout the cardiac cycle. Visual or computer-aided analysis of such images provides information useful in clinically evaluating cardiac function. These techniques are especially suited for detecting abnormal operation of cardiac valves or contractile function in portions of the heart walls. They can also provide estimates of heart chamber volumes at different times in the cardiac cycle that, as described later, are used in a number of ways to assess cardiac function.

Echocardiography is the most widely used of the cardiac imaging techniques currently available. This noninvasive technique is based on the fact that sound waves reflect back toward the source when encountering abrupt changes in the density of the medium through which they travel. A transducer, placed at specified locations on the chest, generates pulses of ultrasonic waves and detects reflected waves that bounce off the cardiac tissue interfaces. The longer the time between the transmission of the wave and the arrival of the reflection, the deeper the structure is in the thorax. Such information can be reconstructed by computer in various ways to produce a continuous image of the heart and its chambers throughout the cardiac cycle.

Cardiac angiography involves the placement of catheters into the right or left ventricle and injection of radiopaque contrast medium during high-speed x-ray filming (cineradiography). *Radionuclide ventriculography* (also known as multigated acquisition scan or MUGA scan) involves the intravenous injection of a radioactive isotope that stays in the vascular space (usually technetium that binds to red blood cells) with measurement of the changes in intensity of radiation detected over the ventricles during the cardiac cycle. A gamma camera is used to obtain images "gated" to different times in the cardiac cycle.

Information derived from the various imaging techniques can be used to evaluate myocardial contractility, a critically important component of cardiac function.

Ejection Fraction

Ejection fraction (EF) is an extremely useful clinical measurement that can be calculated from an echocardiogram. The ejection fraction is defined as the ratio of stroke volume (SV) to end-diastolic volume (EDV):

$$EF = SV/EDV$$

Estimates of end-diastolic and end-systolic volumes can be made from the images and stroke volume calculated. Ejection fraction is commonly expressed as a percentage and normally ranges from 55 to 80% (mean 67%) under resting conditions. Ejection fractions of less than 55% indicate depressed myocardial contractility.

End-Systolic Pressure–Volume Relationship

The end-systolic pressure–volume relationship is useful used clinical technique to assess cardiac contractility. End-systolic volume for a given cardiac cycle is estimated by one of the imaging techniques described previously, while end-systolic pressure for that cardiac cycle can obtained from the arterial pressure record at the point of the closure of the aortic valve (the incisura). Values for several different cardiac cycles may be obtained during infusion of a vasoconstrictor (which increases afterload),

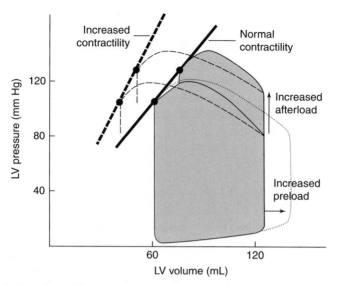

Figure 4–1. The effect of increased contractility on the left ventricular end-systolic pressure–volume relationship.

and the data plotted as in Figure 4–1 in the context of overall ventricular pressure–volume loops. As shown, increases in myocardial contractility are associated with a leftward rotation in the end-systolic pressure–volume relationship. Decreases in contractility (as may be caused by heart disease) are associated with a downward shift of the line, discussed further in Chapter 11. This method of assessing cardiac function is particularly important because it provides an estimate of contractility that is independent of the end-diastolic volume (preload). (Recall from Figure 3–4 and from the pressure–volume loop described by the dotted line in Figure 4–1 that increases in preload cause increases in stroke volume without changing the end-systolic volume. Thus, only alterations in contractility will cause shifts in the end-systolic pressure–volume relationship.)

Note in Figure 4–1 that both the "normal" and "increased contractility" end-systolic pressure–volume lines nearly project to the origin of zero pressure, zero volume. Thus, it is possible to get a reasonable clinical estimate of the slope of the end-systolic pressure–volume relationship (read "myocardial contractility") from a single measurement of end-systolic pressure and volume. This avoids the need to do multiple expensive tests with vasodilator or vasoconstrictor infusions.

MEASUREMENT OF CARDIAC EXCITATION— THE ELECTROCARDIOGRAM

 The electrocardiogram is a powerful clinical tool that is used to evaluate cardiac beating rate, rhythm, and conduction characteristics of cardiac tissue. As briefly described in Chapter 2, the electrocardiogram is the result of

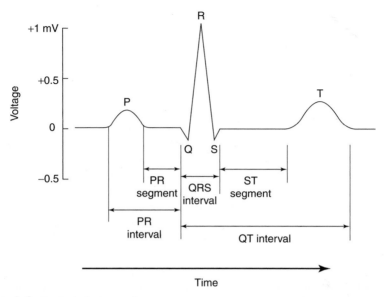

Figure 4–2. Typical electrocardiogram.

currents propagated through the extracellular fluid that are generated by the spread of the wave of excitation throughout the heart. Electrodes placed on the surface of the body record the small potential differences between various recording sites that vary over the time course of the cardiac cycle.

A typical electrocardiographic record is indicated in Figure 4–2. The major features of the electrocardiogram are the P, QRS, and T waves that are caused by atrial depolarization, ventricular depolarization, and ventricular repolarization, respectively. The period from the initiation of the P wave to the beginning of QRS complex is designated as the PR interval and indicates the time it takes for an action potential to spread through the atria and the atrioventricular (AV) node. During the latter portion of the PR interval (PR segment), no voltages are detected on the body surface. This is because atrial muscle cells are depolarized (in the plateau phase of their action potentials), ventricular cells are still resting, and the electrical field setup by the action potential progressing through the small AV node is not intense enough to be detected. The duration of the normal PR interval ranges from 120 to 200 ms. Shortly after the cardiac impulse breaks out of the AV node and into the rapidly conducting Purkinje system, all the ventricular muscle cells depolarize within a very short period and cause the QRS complex. The R wave is the largest event in the electrocardiogram because ventricular muscle cells are so numerous and because they depolarize nearly in unison. The normal QRS complex lasts between 60 and 100 ms. (The repolarization of atrial cells is also occurring during the period in which ventricular depolarization generates the QRS complex on the electrocardiogram, see Figure 2–5. Atrial repolarization is not evident on the electrocardiogram because it is a poorly synchronized event in a relatively small mass of heart tissue and is completely overshadowed by the major electrical events occurring in the ventricles at this time.)

The QRS complex is followed by the *ST segment*. Normally, no electrical potentials are measured on the body surface during the ST segment because no rapid changes in membrane potential are occurring in any of the cells of the heart; atrial cells have already returned to the resting phase, whereas ventricular muscle cells are in the plateau phase of their action potentials. (Myocardial injury or inadequate blood flow, however, can produce elevations or depressions in the ST segment.) When ventricular cells begin to repolarize, a voltage once again appears on the body surface and is measured as the T wave of the electrocardiogram. The T wave is broader and not as large as the R wave because ventricular repolarization is less synchronous than depolarization. At the conclusion of the T wave, all the cells in the heart are in the resting state. The *QT interval* roughly approximates the duration of the ventricular myocyte depolarization and thus the period of ventricular systole. At a normal heart rate of 60 beats per minute, the QT interval is normally less than 380 ms. No body surface potential is measured until the next impulse is generated by the sinoatrial (SA) node.

It should be recognized that the operation of the specialized conduction system is a primary factor in determining the normal electrocardiographic pattern. For example, the AV nodal transmission time determines the PR interval. Also, the effectiveness of the Purkinje system in synchronizing ventricular depolarization is reflected in the large magnitude and short duration of the QRS complex. It should also be noted that nearly every heart muscle cell is inherently capable of rhythmicity and that all cardiac cells are electrically interconnected through gap junctions. Thus, a functional heart rhythm can and often does occur without the involvement of part or all of the specialized conduction system. Such a situation is, however, abnormal, and the existence of abnormal conduction pathways would produce an abnormal electrocardiogram.

Basic Electrocardiographic Conventions

Recording electrocardiograms is a routine diagnostic procedure, which is standardized by universal application of certain conventions. The conventions for recording and analysis of electrocardiograms from the three standard bipolar limb leads are briefly described here.

Recording electrodes are placed on both arms and the left leg—usually at the wrists and ankle. The appendages are assumed to act merely as extensions of the recording system, and voltage measurements are assumed to be made between points that form an equilateral triangle over the thorax, as shown in Figure 4–3. This conceptualization is called *Einthoven's triangle* in honor of the Dutch physiologist who devised it at the turn of the century. Any single electrocardiographic trace is a recording of the voltage difference measured between any two vertices of Einthoven's triangle. An example of the lead II electrocardiogram measured between the right arm and the left leg has already been shown in Figure 4–2. Similarly, lead I and lead III electrocardiograms represent voltage measurements taken along the other

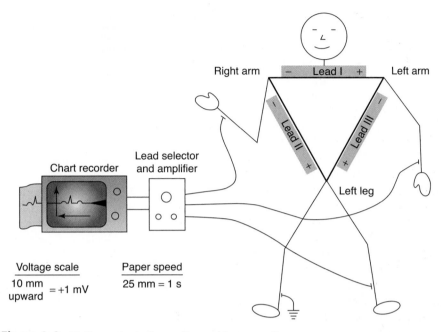

Figure 4–3. Einthoven's electrocardiographic conventions.

two sides of Einthoven's triangle, as indicated in Figure 4–3. The "+" and "−" symbols in Figure 4–3 indicate polarity conventions that have been universally adopted. For example, an upward deflection in a lead II electrocardiogram (as normally occurs during the P, R, and T waves) indicates that an electrical polarity exists at that instant between the left leg and the right shoulder electrodes, with the left leg electrode being positive. Conversely, a downward deflection in a lead II record indicates that a polarity exists between the electrodes at that instant, with the left leg electrode being negative. Similar polarity conventions have been established for lead I and lead III recordings and are indicated by the "+" and "−" symbols in Figure 4–3. In addition, electrocardiographic recording equipment is often standardized so that a 1-cm deflection on the vertical axis always represents a potential difference of 1 mV, and that 25 mm on the horizontal axis of any electrocardiographic record represents 1 second. Most electrocardiographic records contain calibration signals so that abnormal rates and wave amplitudes can be easily detected.

As shown in the next chapter, many cardiac electrical abnormalities can be detected in recordings from a single electrocardiographic lead. However, certain clinically useful information can be derived only by combining the information obtained from two electrocardiographic leads. To understand these more complex electrocardiographic analyses, a close examination of how voltages appear on the body surface as a result of the cardiac electrical activity must be done.

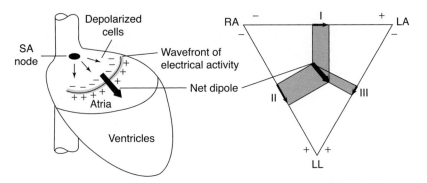

Figure 4–4. Net cardiac dipole during atrial depolarization and its components on the limb leads.

CARDIAC DIPOLES AND ELECTROCARDIOGRAPHIC RECORDS

Einthoven's conceptualization of how cardiac electrical activity causes potential differences on the surface of the body is illustrated in Figure 4–4. In this example, the heart is shown at one instant in the atrial depolarization phase. The cardiac impulse, after having arisen in the SA node, is spreading as a wavefront of depolarization through the atrial tissue. At each point along this wavefront of electrical activity, a small charge separation exists in the extracellular fluid between polarized membranes (positive outside) and depolarized membranes (negative outside). Thus, the wavefront may be thought of as a series of individual *electrical dipoles* (regions of charge separation). Each individual dipole is oriented in the direction of local wavefront movement. The large, black arrow in Figure 4–4 represents the total *net* dipole created by the summed contributions of all the individual dipoles distributed along the wavefront of atrial depolarization. The salty extracellular fluid acts as an excellent conductor, allowing these instantaneous net dipoles, generated on the surface of the heart muscle to be recorded by electrodes on the surface of the body.

The net dipole that exists at any instant is oriented (ie, points) in the general direction of wavefront movement at that instant. The magnitude or strength of the dipole (represented here by the arrow length) is determined by (1) how extensive the wavefront is (ie, how many cells are simultaneously depolarizing at the instant in question) and (2) the consistency of orientation between individual dipoles at different points in the wavefront (dipoles with the same orientation reinforce each other; dipoles with opposite orientation cancel each other).

The net dipole in the example in Figure 4–4 causes the lower-left portion of the body to be generally positive with respect to the upper-right portion. This particular dipole will cause positive voltages to exist on all three of the electrocardiogram limb leads. As shown in the right half of Figure 4–4, this can be deduced from Einthoven's triangle by observing that the net dipole has some component that points in the positive direction of leads I, II, and III. As illustrated in Figure 4–4, the component that a cardiac dipole has on a given electrocardiogram lead is found by drawing perpendicular lines from the appropriate side of Einthoven's triangle to the tip and tail of the dipole. (It may be helpful to think of the component on each lead as the "shadow" cast by the dipole on that lead as a result of a "sun" located far beyond the corner of Einthoven's triangle that is opposite the lead.) Note that the dipole in this example is most parallel to lead II and therefore has a large component in the lead II direction. Thus, it will create a larger voltage on lead II than on lead I or III. This dipole has a rather small component on lead III because it is oriented nearly perpendicular to lead III.

The limb lead configuration may be thought of as a way to view the heart's electrical activity from three different perspectives (or axes). The vector representing the heart's instantaneous dipole strength and orientation is the object under observation, and its appearance depends on the position from which it is viewed. The instantaneous voltage measured on the axis of lead I, for example, indicates how the dipole being generated by the heart's electrical activity at that instant appears when viewed from directly above. A cardiac dipole that is oriented horizontally appears large on lead I, whereas a vertically oriented cardiac dipole, however large, produces no voltage on lead I. Thus, it is necessary to have views from two directions to establish the magnitude and orientation of the heart's dipole. A vertically oriented dipole would be invisible on lead I but would be readily apparent if viewed from the perspective of lead II or lead III.

It is important to recognize that the example in Figure 4–4 pertains only to one instant during atrial depolarization. The net cardiac dipole continually changes in magnitude and orientation during the course of atrial depolarization. The nature of these changes will determine the shape of the P wave on each of the electrocardiogram leads.

The P wave terminates when the wave of depolarization, as illustrated in Figure 4–4, reaches the nonmuscular border between the atria and the ventricles and the number of individual dipoles becomes very small. At this time, the cardiac impulse is still being slowly transmitted toward the ventricles through the AV node. However, the electrical activity in the AV node involves so few cells that it generates no detectable net cardiac dipole. Thus, no voltages are measured on the surface of the body for a brief period following the P wave. A net cardiac dipole reappears only when the depolarization completes its passage through the AV node, enters the Purkinje system, and begins its rapid passage over the ventricular muscle cells. Because the Purkinje fibers initially pass through the intraventricular septum and to the endocardial layers at the apex of the ventricles, ventricular depolarization occurs first in these areas and then proceeds outward and upward through the ventricular myocardium.

Ventricular Depolarization and the QRS Complex

It is the rapid and large changes in the magnitude and direction of the net cardiac dipole that occur during ventricular depolarization that cause the QRS complex of the electrocardiogram. The normal process is illustrated in Figure 4–5. The

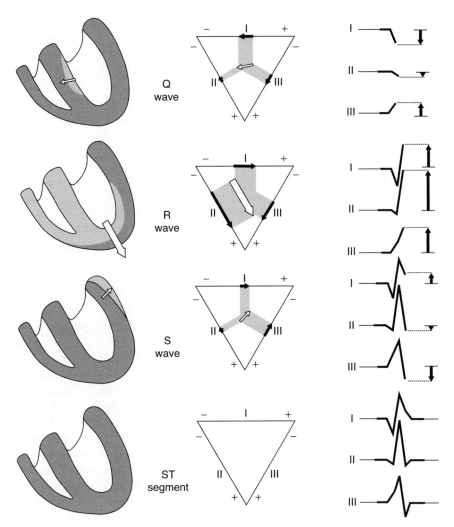

Figure 4–5. Ventricular depolarization and the generation of the QRS complex.

initial ventricular depolarization usually occurs on the left side of the intraventricular septum as illustrated in the upper panel of the figure. Analysis of the cardiac dipole formed by this initial ventricular depolarization with the aid of Einthoven's triangle shows that this dipole has a negative component on lead I, a small negative component on lead II, and a positive component on lead III. The upper right panel shows the actual deflections on each of the electrocardiographic limb leads that will be produced by this dipole. Note that it is possible for a given cardiac dipole to produce opposite deflections on different leads. For example, in Figure 4–5, Q waves appear on leads I and II but not on lead III.

The second row of panels in Figure 4–5 shows the ventricles during the instant in ventricular depolarization when the number of individual dipoles is greatest and/or their orientation is most similar. This phase generates the large net cardiac dipole, which is responsible for the R wave of the electrocardiogram. In Figure 4–5, this net cardiac dipole is nearly parallel to lead II. As indicated, such a dipole produces large positive R waves on all three limb leads.

The third row in Figure 4–5 shows the situation near the end of the spread of depolarization through the ventricles and indicates how the small net cardiac dipole present at this time produces the S wave. Note that an S wave does not necessarily appear on all electrocardiogram leads (as in lead I of this example).

The bottom row in Figure 4–5 shows that during the ST segment, all ventricular muscle cells are in a depolarized state. There are no waves of electrical activity moving through the heart tissue. Consequently, no net cardiac dipole exists at this time and no voltage differences exist between points on the body surface. All electrocardiographic traces will be flat at the *isoelectric* (zero voltage) level.

Ventricular Repolarization and the T Wave

As illustrated in Figure 4–2, the T wave is normally positive on lead II as is the R wave. This indicates that the net cardiac dipole generated during ventricular repolarization is oriented in the same general direction as that which exists during ventricular depolarization. This may be somewhat surprising. However, recall from Figure 2–5 that the *last ventricular cells to depolarize are the first to repolarize*. The reasons for this are not well understood, but the result is that the wavefront of electrical activity during ventricular repolarization tends to retrace, in *reverse direction*, the course followed during ventricular depolarization. Therefore, the dipole formed during repolarization has the *same* polarity as that during depolarization. This reversed wavefront propagation pathway during ventricular repolarization results in a positive T wave recorded, for example, on lead II. The T wave is broader and smaller than the R wave because the repolarization of ventricular muscle cells is less well synchronized than is their depolarization.

MEAN ELECTRICAL AXIS AND AXIS DEVIATIONS

The orientation of the cardiac dipole during the most intense phase of ventricular depolarization (ie, at the instant the R wave reaches its peak) is called the *mean electrical axis* of the heart. It is used clinically as an indicator of whether ventricular depolarization is proceeding over normal pathways. The mean electrical axis is reported in degrees according to the convention indicated in Figure 4–6. (Note that the downward direction corresponds to *plus* 90 degrees in this polar coordinate system.) As indicated, a mean electrical axis that lies anywhere in the patient's lower left-hand quadrant is considered normal. A *left axis deviation* exists when the mean electrical axis falls in the patient's upper left-hand quadrant and may indicate a physical displacement of the heart to the left, left ventricular hypertrophy, or loss of electrical activity in the right ventricle. A *right axis deviation*

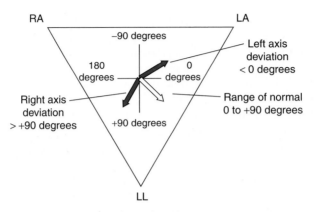

Figure 4–6. Mean electrical axis and axis deviations.

exists when the mean electrical axis falls in the patient's lower right-hand quadrant and may indicate a physical displacement of the heart to the right, right ventricular hypertrophy, or loss of electrical activity in the left ventricle.

The mean electrical axis of the heart can be determined from the electrocardiogram. The process involves determining what single net dipole orientation will produce the R-wave amplitudes recorded on any two leads. For example, if the R waves on leads II and III are both positive (upright) and of equal magnitude, the mean electrical axis must be +90 degrees. As should be obvious, in this case, the amplitude of the R wave on lead I will be zero.[1] Alternatively, one can scan the electrocardiographic records for the lead tracing with the largest R waves and then deduce that the mean electrical axis must be nearly parallel to that lead. In Figure 4–5, for example, the largest R wave occurs on lead II. Lead II has an orientation of +60 degrees, which is very close to the actual mean electrical axis in this example.

Another analysis technique called *vectorcardiography* is based on continuously following the magnitude and orientation of the heart's dipole throughout the cardiac cycle. A typical vectorcardiogram is illustrated in Figure 4–7 and is a graphical record of the dipole amplitude in the x and y directions throughout a single cardiac cycle. If one imagines the heart's electrical dipole as a vector with its tail always positioned at the center of Einthoven's triangle, then the vectorcardiogram can be thought of as a complete record of all the various positions that the head of the dipole assumes during the course of one cardiac cycle. A vectorcardiogram starts from an isoelectric diastolic point and traces three loops during each cardiac

---

[1] An accurate, albeit tedious, way to determine the mean electrical axis is to follow these steps: (1) determine the algebraic sum of the R- and S-wave amplitude on each of the two leads, (2) plot these magnitudes as components on the appropriate sides of Einthoven's equilateral triangle according to the standardized polarity conventions, (3) project perpendicular lines from the heads and tails of these components into the interior of the triangle to find the position of the head and tail of the cardiac dipole, which produced the R waves, and (4) measure the angular orientation of this dipole.

Figure 4–7. Typical vectorcardiogram.

cycle. The first small loop is caused by atrial depolarization, the second large loop is caused by ventricular depolarization, and the final intermediate-sized loop is caused by ventricular repolarization. The mean electrical axis of the ventricle is immediately apparent in a vectorcardiographic record as the orientation of the largest deviation from the isoelectric point during ventricular depolarization. Analogous "mean axes" can similarly be defined for the P wave and T wave but are not commonly used.

THE STANDARD 12-LEAD ELECTROCARDIOGRAM

The standard clinical electrocardiogram involves voltage measurements recorded from 12 different leads. Three of these are the bipolar limb leads I, II, and III, which have already been discussed. The other 9 leads are unipolar leads. Three of these leads are generated by using the limb electrodes. Two of the electrodes are electrically connected to form an *indifferent electrode*, while the third limb electrode is made the positive pole of the pair. Recordings made from these electrodes are called *augmented unipolar limb leads*. The voltage record obtained between the electrode on the right arm and the indifferent electrode is called a lead aVR electrocardiogram. Similarly, lead aVL is recorded from the electrode on the left arm, and lead aVF is recorded from the electrode on the left leg.

The standard limb leads (I, II, and III) and the augmented unipolar limb leads (aVR, aVL, and aVF) record the electrical activity of the heart as it appears from six different "perspectives," all in the frontal plane. As shown in Figure 4–8A, the axes for leads I, II, and III are those of the sides of Einthoven's triangle, while those for aVR, aVL, and aVF are specified by lines drawn from the center of Einthoven's triangle to each of its vertices. As indicated in Figure 4–8B, these six limb leads can be thought of as a hexaxial reference system for observing the cardiac vectors in the frontal plane.

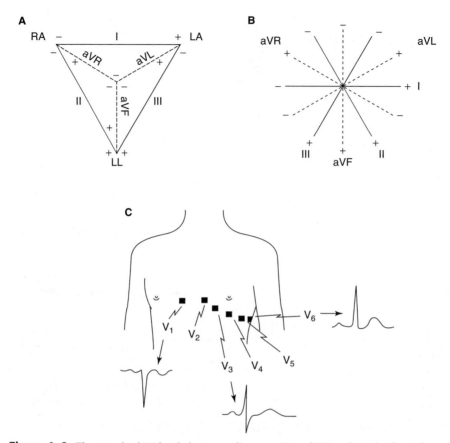

Figure 4–8. The standard 12-lead electrocardiogram. (**A** and **B**) Leads in the frontal plane. (**C**) Electrode positions for precordial leads in the transverse plane.

The other six leads of the standard 12-lead electrocardiogram are also unipolar leads that "look" at the electrical vector projections in the transverse plane. These potentials are obtained by placing an additional (*exploring*) electrode in six specified positions on the chest wall as shown in Figure 4–8C. The indifferent electrode in this case is formed by electrically connecting the limb electrodes. These leads are identified as *precordial* or *chest* leads and are designated as V1 through V6. As shown in this figure, when the positive electrode is placed in position 1 and the wave of ventricular excitation sweeps away from it, the resultant deflection will be downward. When the electrode is in position 6 and the wave of ventricular excitation sweeps toward it, the deflection will be upward.

In summary, the electrocardiogram is a powerful tool for evaluating cardiac excitation characteristics. It must be recognized, however, that the ECG does not provide direct evidence of mechanical pumping effectiveness. For example, a leaky valve will have no direct electrocardiographic consequences but may adversely influence pumping ability of the heart.

KEY CONCEPTS

 A variety of methods are available for measuring various aspects of cardiac mechanical function. These methods are based on the Fick principle, dye-dilution techniques, and various imaging techniques including echocardiography.

 The ejection fraction (stroke volume/end-diastolic volume) is a very useful index of cardiac contractility.

 The electrocardiogram is a record of the voltage changes that occur on the surface of the body as a result of the propagation of the action potential through the heart during a cardiac cycle.

 There are standardized conventions used for recording electrocardiograms.

 The magnitude and direction of the net dipole formed by the wavefront of the action potential at any instant in time can be deduced from the magnitude and orientation of the electrocardiographic deflections.

 The mean electrical axis describes the orientation of the net dipole at the instant of maximum wavefront propagation during ventricular depolarization and normally falls between 0 and +90 degrees on a polar coordinate system.

 The standard 12-lead electrocardiogram is widely used to evaluate cardiac electrical activity and consists of a combination of bipolar and unipolar records from limb electrodes and chest electrodes.

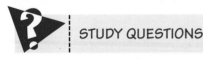 STUDY QUESTIONS

4–1. Given the following information, calculate cardiac output:

Systemic arterial blood oxygen concentration, $[O_2]_{SA} = 200$ mL/L
Pulmonary arterial blood oxygen concentration, $[O_2]_{PA} = 140$ mL/L
Total body oxygen consumption, $VO_2 = 600$ mL/min

4–2. If left ventricular end-diastolic volume is 150 mL and end-systolic volume is 50 mL, what is the ejection fraction? Is this "normal" for a resting adult?

4–3. A decrease in atrioventricular nodal conduction velocity will

a. decrease the heart rate
b. increase P-wave amplitude
c. increase the PR interval
d. widen the QRS complex
e. increase the ST-segment duration

4–4. The P wave on lead aVR of the normal electrocardiogram will be

    a. an upward deflection

    b. a downward deflection

    c. not detectable

    d. highly variable

4–5. If the R wave is upright and equally large on leads I and aVF, what is the mean electrical axis of the heart? Is it within normal range? Which lead(s) will have the smallest R wave amplitude?

4–6. What is the definition of cardiac "ejection fraction"?

    a. stroke volume expressed as a percent of cardiac output

    b. the ratio of the end-systolic volume to the end-diastolic volume

    c. the ratio of the end-diastolic volume to the end-systolic volume

    d. the ratio of stroke volume to the end-diastolic volume

    e. the ratio of the time spent in systole to the time spent in diastole

4–7. Electrocardiograms give information about all of the following except

    a. atrial beating rate

    b. site of pacemaker origination

    c. pathway of ventricular activation

    d. rate of AV nodal conduction

    e. amplitude of the ventricular action potential

4–8. If something slows the conduction pathway of the action potential through the ventricular muscle, which of the following alterations would you most likely see on the ECG?

    a. absence of P waves

    b. prolongation of the PR interval

    c. prolongation of the QRS interval

    d. shortening of the QT interval

    e. elevation of the ST segment

Cardiac Abnormalities 5

OBJECTIVES

The student, through understanding normal cardiac function, diagnoses and appreciates the consequences of common cardiac abnormalities:

▶ *Detects common cardiac arrhythmias from the electrocardiogram, identifies their physiological bases, and describes their physiological consequences.*

▶ *Lists four common valvular abnormalities for the left side of the heart and describes the alterations in intracardiac and arterial pressures, flow patterns, and heart sounds that accompany them.*

Recall that effective, efficient ventricular pumping action depends on proper cardiac function in five basic aspects. This chapter focuses on the abnormalities in three of these aspects: (1) abnormal cardiac excitation and rhythmicity, (2) valvular stenosis (inadequate valve opening), and (3) valvular insufficiency (incomplete valve closure). Discussion of abnormalities in myocardial force production and cardiac filling is presented in Chapter 11. The material presented here is an introduction to the more common cardiac electrical and valvular dysfunctions, with an emphasis on the primary physiological consequences of these abnormal situations.

ELECTRICAL ABNORMALITIES AND ARRHYTHMIAS

Many cardiac excitation problems can be diagnosed from the information in a single lead of an electrocardiogram. The lead II electrocardiogram traces at the top of Figure 5–1 and 5–2 are identified as normal sinus rhythms based on the following characteristics: (1) the frequency of QRS complexes is approximately 1 per second, indicating a normal beating rate; (2) the shape of the QRS complex is normal for lead II and its duration is less than 120 ms, indicating rapid depolarization of the ventricles via normal conduction pathways; (3) each QRS complex is preceded by a P wave of proper configuration, indicating sinoatrial (SA) nodal origin of the excitation; (4) the PR interval is less than 200 ms, indicating proper conduction delay of the impulse propagation through the atrioventricular (AV) node; (5) the QT interval is less than half of the R-to-R interval, indicating normal

Figure 5–1. Supraventricular arrhythmias.

ventricular repolarization; and (6) there are no extra P waves, indicating that no AV nodal conduction block is present. The subsequent electrocardiographic tracings in Figures 5–1 and 5–2 represent irregularities commonly found in clinical practice. Examination of each of these traces with the above characteristics in mind will aid in the differential diagnosis.

Figure 5–2. Ventricular arrhythmias.

The physiological consequences of abnormal excitation and conduction in the heart depend on whether the electrical abnormality evokes a *tachycardia*, which will limit the time for cardiac filling between beats; evokes a *bradycardia*, which is inadequate to support sufficient cardiac output; or decreases the coordination of myocyte contraction, which will reduce stroke volume.

Supraventricular Abnormalities

Traces 2 through 6 below the normal trace in Figure 5–1 represent typical supraventricular arrhythmias (ie, originating in the atria or AV node). *Supraventricular tachycardia* (shown in trace 2 in Figure 5–1 and sometimes called *paroxysmal atrial tachycardia*) occurs when the atria are abnormally excited and drive the ventricles at a very rapid rate. These paroxysms begin abruptly, last for a few minutes to a few hours, and then, just as abruptly, disappear and the heart rate reverts to normal. QRS complexes appear normal (albeit frequent) with simple paroxysmal atrial tachycardia because the ventricular conduction pathways operate normally. The P and T waves may be superimposed because of the high heart rate. Low blood pressure and dizziness may accompany bouts of this arrhythmia because the extremely high heart rate does not allow sufficient diastolic time for ventricular filling.

There are two mechanisms that may account for supraventricular tachycardia. First, an atrial region, usually outside the SA node, may become irritable (perhaps because of local interruption in blood flow) and begin to fire rapidly to take over the pacemaker function. Such an abnormal pacemaker region is called an *ectopic focus*. Alternatively, atrial conduction may become altered so that a single wave of excitation does not die out but continually travels around some abnormal atrial conduction loop. In this case, the continual activity in the conduction loop may drive the atria and AV node at a very high frequency. This self-sustaining process is called a *reentry phenomenon* and is illustrated in Figure 5–3. This situation

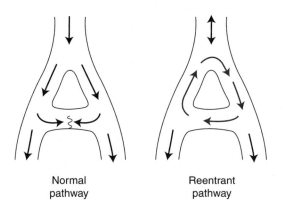

Normal
pathway

Reentrant
pathway

Figure 5–3. Normal and reentrant (circus) cardiac excitation pathways.

may develop as a result of abnormal repolarization and altered refractory periods in local areas of the myocardium. *Atrial flutter* is a special form of tachycardia of atrial origin in which a large reentrant pathway drives the atria at very fast rates (250 to 300 beats per minute) and normal refractory periods of AV nodal tissue are overwhelmed. Thus, ventricular rate is often some fixed ratio of the atrial rate (2:1, 4:1) with frequencies often 150 to 220 beats per minute. The electrocardiogram often shows a sawtooth pattern of merged P waves with intermittent normal QRS complexes.

 Conduction blocks occur at the AV node and generally represent impaired conduction through this tissue. In a *first-degree heart block* (trace 3 in Figure 5–1), the only electrical abnormality is unusually slow conduction through the AV node. This condition is detected by an abnormally long PR interval (>0.2 second). Otherwise, the electrocardiogram may be completely normal. At normal heart rates, the physiological effects of the first-degree block are inconsequential. The danger, however, is that the slow conduction may deteriorate to an actual interruption of conduction.

A *second-degree heart block* (trace 4 in Figure 5–1) is said to exist when some but not all atrial impulses are transmitted through the AV node to the ventricle. Impulses are blocked in the AV node if the cells of the region are still in a refractory period from a previous excitation. The situation is aggravated by high atrial rates and slower than normal conduction through the AV nodal region. In the second-degree block, some but not all P waves are accompanied by corresponding QRS complexes and T waves. Atrial rate is often faster than ventricular rate by a certain ratio (eg, 2:1, 3:1, and 4:1). This condition may not represent a serious clinical problem as long as the ventricular rate is adequate to meet the pumping needs.

In a *third-degree heart block* (trace 5 in Figure 5–1), no impulses are transmitted through the AV node. In this event, some area in the ventricles—often in the common bundle or bundle branches near the exit of the AV node—assumes the pacemaker role for the ventricular tissue. Atrial rate and ventricular rate are completely independent, and P waves and QRS complexes are totally dissociated in the electrocardiogram. Ventricular rate is likely to be slower than normal (bradycardia) and sometimes is slow enough to impair cardiac output.

Atrial fibrillation (trace 6 in Figure 5–1) is characterized by a complete loss of the normally close synchrony of the excitation and resting phases between individual atrial cells. Cells in different areas of the atria depolarize, repolarize, and are excited again randomly. Consequently, no P waves appear in the electrocardiogram although there may be rapid, irregular, small waves apparent throughout diastole. The ventricular rate is often very irregular in atrial fibrillation because impulses enter the AV node from the atria at unpredictable times. Fibrillation is a self-sustaining process. The mechanisms behind it are not well understood, but impulses are thought to progress repeatedly around irregular conduction pathways (sometimes called circus pathways, which imply a reentry phenomenon as described earlier and in Figure 5–3). However, because atrial contraction usually plays a negligible role in ventricular filling, atrial fibrillation may be well tolerated by most patients as long as ventricular rate is sufficient to maintain the cardiac output.[1]

Ventricular Abnormalities

 Traces 2 through 6 below the normal trace in Figure 5–2 show typical ventricular electrical abnormalities. Conduction blocks called *bundle branch blocks* or *hemiblocks* (trace 2 in Figure 5–2) can occur in either of the branches of the Purkinje system of the intraventricular septum often as a result of a myocardial infarction. Ventricular depolarization is less synchronous than normal in the half of the heart with the nonfunctional Purkinje system. This results in a widening of the QRS complex (>0.12 second) because a longer time is required for ventricular depolarization to be completed. The direct physiological effects of bundle branch blocks are usually inconsequential.

Premature ventricular contractions (PVCs) (trace 3 in Figure 5–2) are caused by action potentials initiated by and propagated away from an ectopic focus in the ventricle. As a result, the ventricle depolarizes and contracts before it normally would. A PVC is often followed by a missed beat (called a *compensatory pause*) because the ventricular cells are still refractory when the next normal impulse emerges from the SA node. The highly abnormal ventricular depolarization pattern of a PVC produces the large-amplitude, long-duration deflections on the electrocardiogram. The shapes of the electrocardiographic records of these extra beats are highly variable and depend on the ectopic site of their origin and the depolarization pathways involved. The volume of blood ejected by the premature beat itself is smaller than normal, whereas the stroke volume of the beat following the compensatory pause is larger than normal. This is partly due to the differences in filling times and partly to an inherent phenomenon of the cardiac muscle called *postextrasystolic potentiation.* Single PVCs occur occasionally in most individuals and, although sometimes alarming to the individual experiencing them, are not dangerous. Frequent occurrence of PVCs, however, may be a signal of possible myocardial damage or perfusion problems.

Ventricular tachycardia (trace 4 in Figure 5–2) occurs when the ventricles are driven at high rates, usually by impulses originating from a ventricular ectopic focus. Ventricular tachycardia is a very serious condition. Not only is diastolic filling time limited by the rapid rate, but the abnormal excitation pathways make ventricular contraction less synchronous and therefore less effective than normal. In addition, ventricular tachycardia often precedes ventricular fibrillation.

Prolonged QT intervals (the left side of trace 5 in Figure 5–2) are a result of delayed ventricular myocyte repolarization, which may be due to inappropriate opening of

---

[1] The real danger with atrial fibrillation lies in the tendency for blood to form clots in the atria in the absence of the normal vigorous coordinated atrial contraction. These clots can fragment and move out of the heart to lodge in small arteries throughout the systemic circulation. These emboli can have devastating effects on critical organ function. Consequently, anticoagulant therapy is usually prescribed for patients in atrial fibrillation.

sodium channels or prolonged closure of potassium channels during the action potential plateau phase. Although the normal QT interval varies with heart rate, it is normally less than 40% of the cardiac cycle length (except at very high heart rates). Long QT syndrome is identified when the QT interval is greater than 50% of the cycle duration. It may be genetic in origin (mutations influencing various ion channels involved with cardiac excitability), may be acquired from several electrolyte disturbances (low blood levels of Ca^{2+}, Mg^{2+}, or K^+), or may be induced by several pharmacological agents (including some antiarrhythmic drugs). The prolongation of the myocyte refractory period, which accompanies the long QT syndrome, extends the vulnerable period during which extra stimuli can evoke tachycardia or fibrillation. Patients with long QT syndrome are predisposed to a particularly dangerous type of ventricular tachycardia called *torsades de pointes* ("twisting of points" as shown in the right side of trace 5 in Figure 5–2). This differs from the ordinary ventricular tachycardia in that the ventricular electrical complexes cyclically vary in amplitude around the baseline and can deteriorate rapidly into ventricular fibrillation.

In *ventricular fibrillation* (trace 6 in Figure 5–2), various areas of the ventricle are excited and contract asynchronously. The mechanisms are similar to those in atrial fibrillation. The ventricle is especially susceptible to fibrillation whenever a premature excitation occurs at the end of the T wave of the previous excitation, that is, when most ventricular cells are in the "hyperexcitable" or "vulnerable" period of their electrical cycle. In addition, because some cells are repolarized and some are still refractory, circus pathways can be triggered easily at this time. Since no pumping action occurs with ventricular fibrillation, the situation is fatal unless quickly corrected by *cardiac conversion*. During conversion, the artificial application of large currents to the entire heart (via paddle electrodes applied across the chest) may be effective in depolarizing all heart cells simultaneously and thus allowing a normal excitation pathway to be reestablished.

VALVULAR ABNORMALITIES

Pumping action of the heart is impaired when the valves do not function properly. Abnormal heart sounds, which usually accompany cardiac valvular defects, are called *murmurs*. These sounds are caused by abnormal pressure gradients and turbulent blood flow patterns that occur during the cardiac cycle. A number of techniques, ranging from simple auscultation (listening to the heart sounds) to echocardiography or cardiac catheterization, are used to obtain information about the nature and extent of these valvular malfunctions.

In general, when a valve does not open fully (ie, is stenotic), the chamber upstream of the valve has to develop more pressure during its systolic phase to achieve a given flow through the valve. This increase in "pressure" work will induce hypertrophy of cardiac muscle cells and thickening of the walls of that chamber. When a valve does not close completely (ie, is insufficient), the regurgitant blood flow represents an additional volume that must be ejected in order to get sufficient forward flow out of the ventricle into the tissues. This increase in "volume" work often leads to chamber dilation but not to an increase in wall thickness.[2]

A second generality about valve abnormalities is that whenever there is an elevation in the atrial pressure as a result of AV valve stenosis or regurgitation, this will result in higher pressures in the upstream capillary beds. If capillary hydrostatic pressures are elevated, tissue edema will ensue with consequences on the function of those upstream organs.

A brief overview of four of the common valve defects influencing left ventricular function is given in Figure 5–4. Note that similar stenotic and regurgitant abnormalities can occur in right ventricular valves with similar consequences on right ventricular function.

Aortic Stenosis

Some characteristics of aortic stenosis are shown in Figure 5–4A. Normally, the aortic valve opens widely and offers a pathway of very low resistance through which blood leaves the left ventricle. If this opening is narrowed (stenotic), resistance to flow through the valve increases. A significant pressure difference between the left ventricle and the aorta may be required to eject blood through a stenotic aortic valve. As shown in Figure 5–4A, intraventricular pressures may rise to very high levels during systole while aortic pressure rises more slowly than normal to a systolic value that is subnormal. Pulse pressure is usually low with aortic stenosis. High intraventricular pressure development is a strong stimulus for cardiac muscle cell hypertrophy, and an increase in left ventricular muscle mass invariably accompanies aortic stenosis. This tends to produce a leftward deviation of the electrical axis. (The mean electrical axis will fall in the upper right-hand quadrant in Figure 4–6.) Blood being ejected through the narrowed orifice may reach very high velocities, and turbulent flow may occur as blood enters the aorta. This abnormal turbulent flow can be heard as a *systolic* (or ejection) *murmur* with a properly placed stethoscope. The primary physiological consequence of aortic stenosis is a high ventricular afterload that is caused by restriction of the outflow tract. This imposes an increased pressure workload on the left ventricle.

Mitral Stenosis

Some characteristics of mitral stenosis are shown in Figure 5–4B. A pressure difference of more than a few millimeters of mercury across the mitral valve during diastole is distinctly abnormal and indicates that this valve is stenotic. The high resistance mandates an elevated pressure difference to achieve normal flow across the valve ($\dot{Q} = \Delta P/R$). Consequently, as shown in Figure 5–4B, left atrial pressure is elevated with mitral stenosis. The high left atrial workload may induce

---

[2] A useful analogy is to compare the hypertrophied skeletal muscles of the weightlifter (doing isometric or pressure work) to the nonhypertrophied but well-toned skeletal muscles of the long-distance runner (doing isotonic or shortening work).

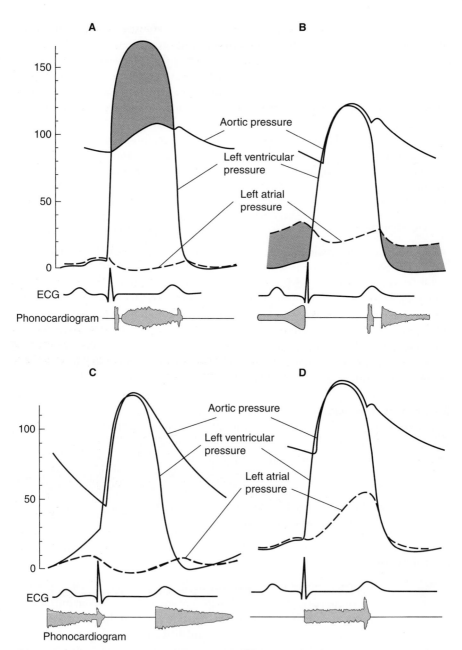

A

150 —
100 —
50 —
0 —

Aortic pressure

Left ventricular pressure

Left atrial pressure

ECG

Phonocardiogram

B

C

100 —
50 —
0 —

Aortic pressure

Left ventricular pressure

Left atrial pressure

ECG

Phonocardiogram

D

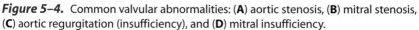

Figure 5–4. Common valvular abnormalities: (**A**) aortic stenosis, (**B**) mitral stenosis, (**C**) aortic regurgitation (insufficiency), and (**D**) mitral insufficiency.

hypertrophy of the left atrial muscle. Elevated left atrial pressure is reflected back into the pulmonary bed and, if high enough, causes pulmonary congestion and "shortness of breath." A *diastolic murmur* associated with turbulent flow through the stenotic mitral valve can often be heard. The primary physiological consequences of mitral stenosis are elevations in left atrial pressure and pulmonary capillary pressure. The latter can cause pulmonary edema and interference with normal gas exchange in the lungs (leading to shortness of breath).

Aortic Insufficiency

Typical characteristics of aortic regurgitation (insufficiency, incompetence) are shown in Figure 5–4C. When the leaflets of the aortic valve do not provide an adequate seal, blood regurgitates from the aorta back into the left ventricle during the diastolic period. Aortic pressure falls faster and further than normal during diastole, which causes a low diastolic pressure and a large pulse pressure. In addition, ventricular end-diastolic volume and pressure are higher than normal because of the extra blood that reenters the chamber through the incompetent aortic valve during diastole. Turbulent flow of the blood reentering the left ventricle during early diastole produces a characteristic diastolic murmur. Often the aortic valve is altered so that it is both stenotic and insufficient. In these instances, both a systolic and a diastolic murmurs are present. The primary physiological consequences of aortic insufficiency are a reduction in forward flow out to the tissues (if the insufficiency is severe) and an increase in the volume workload of the left ventricle.

Mitral Regurgitation

Typical characteristics of mitral regurgitation (insufficiency, incompetence) are shown in Figure 5–4D. When the mitral valve is insufficient, some blood regurgitates from the left ventricle into the left atrium during systole. A systolic murmur may accompany this abnormal flow pattern. Left atrial pressure is raised to abnormally high levels, and left ventricular end-diastolic volume and pressure increase. Mitral valve *prolapse* is a common form of mitral insufficiency in which the valve leaflets evert into the left atrium during systole. The primary physiological consequences of mitral regurgitation are somewhat similar to aortic insufficiency in that forward flow out of the left ventricle into the aorta may be compromised (if the insufficiency is severe) and there is an increase in the volume workload of the left ventricle. In addition, the elevated left atrial pressure can also lead to pulmonary effects with shortness of breath.

KEY CONCEPTS

Cardiac arrhythmias can often be detected and diagnosed from a single electrocardiographic lead.

Physiological consequences of abnormal excitation and conduction in the heart depend on whether the electrical abnormality limits the time for adequate cardiac filling or decreases the coordination of myocyte contractions resulting in inadequate pressure development and ejection.

 Supraventricular arrhythmias are a result of abnormal action potential initiation at the SA node or altered propagation characteristics through the atrial tissue and the AV node.

 Tachycardias may originate either in the atria or in the ventricles and are a result of increased pacemaker automaticity or of continuously circling pathways setting up a reentrant circuit.

 Abnormal conduction through the AV node results in conduction blocks.

 Abnormal conduction pathways in the Purkinje system or in the ventricular tissue result in significant QRS alterations.

 Ventricular tachycardia and ventricular fibrillation represent severe abnormalities that are incompatible with effective cardiac pumping.

 Failure of cardiac valves to open fully (stenosis) can result in elevated upstream chamber pressure and abnormal pressure gradients, congestion in upstream vascular beds, chamber wall hypertrophy, turbulent forward flow across the valve, and murmurs during systole or diastole.

 Failure of cardiac valves to close completely (insufficiency, incompetence, regurgitation) can result in large stroke volumes, abnormal pressure pulses, congestion in upstream vascular beds, turbulent backward flow across the valve, and murmurs during systole or diastole.

STUDY QUESTIONS

5–1. Which of the following arrhythmias might result in a reduced stroke volume?
   a. paroxysmal atrial tachycardia
   b. ventricular tachycardia
   c. atrial fibrillation
   d. ventricular fibrillation
   e. third-degree heart block
5–2. Describe the primary pressure abnormalities associated with
   a. aortic stenosis
   b. mitral stenosis

5–3. You notice an abnormally large pulsation of your patient's jugular vein, which occurs at about the same time as heart sound, S_1. What is your diagnosis?

5–4. What alteration in jugular venous pulsations might accompany third-degree heart block?

5–5. Given the following data, calculate the resistance to flow across this stenotic valve.

Aortic pressures (systolic/diastolic) = 150/100 mmHg

Left ventricular pressures (systolic/diastolic) = 150/2 mmHg

Left atrial pressures (systolic/diastolic) = 50/32 mmHg

Heart rate = 60 beats per minute

Stroke volume = 50 mL/beat

   a. 3.0 L/min

   b. 6.0 L/min

   c. 100 mmHg

   d. 30 mmHg/L per minute

   e. 10 mmHg/L per minute

5–6. Your 75-year-old male patient is alert with complaints of general fatigue. His heart rate = 90 beats per minute and arterial pressure = 180/50 mmHg. A diastolic murmur is present. There are no ECG abnormalities identified and mean electrical axis = 10 degrees. Cardiac catheterization indicates that LV pressure = 180/20 mmHg and left atrial pressure = 10/3 mmHg (as peak systolic/end-diastolic). Which of the following is most consistent with these findings?

   a. aortic stenosis

   b. aortic insufficiency

   c. mitral stenosis

   d. mitral insufficiency

   e. right ventricular hypertrophy

5–7. Evaluation of your patient's electrocardiogram shows that P waves occur at a regular rate of 90 per minute and QRS complexes occur at a regular rate of 37 per minute. Which of the following is the most likely diagnosis?

   a. supraventricular tachycardia

   b. first-degree heart block

   c. second-degree heart block

   d. third-degree heart block

   e. bundle branch block

The Peripheral Vascular System 6

OBJECTIVES

The student understands the basic principles of cardiovascular transport and its role in maintaining homeostasis:

▶ Defines convective transport and diffusion and lists the factors that determine the rate of each.

▶ Given data, uses the Fick principle to calculate the rate of removal of a solute from blood as it passes through an organ.

▶ Describes how capillary wall permeability to a solute is related to the size and lipid solubility of the solute.

▶ Lists the factors that influence transcapillary fluid movement and, given data, predicts the direction of transcapillary fluid movement.

▶ Describes the lymphatic vessel system and its role in preventing fluid accumulation in the interstitial space.

The student understands the physical factors that regulate blood flow through and blood volume in the various components of the vasculature:

▶ Given data, calculates the vascular resistances of networks of vessels arranged in parallel and in series.

▶ Describes differences in the blood flow velocity in the various segments and how these differences are related to their total cross-sectional area.

▶ Describes laminar and turbulent flow patterns and the origin of flow sounds in the cardiovascular system.

▶ Identifies the approximate percentage of the total blood volume that is contained in the various vascular segments in the systemic circulation.

▶ Defines peripheral venous pool and central venous pool.

▶ Describes the pressure changes that occur as blood flows through a vascular bed and relates them to the vascular resistance of the various vascular segments.

▶ States how the resistance of each consecutive vascular segment contributes to an organ's overall vascular resistance and, given data, calculates the overall resistance.

▶ Defines total peripheral resistance (systemic vascular resistance) and states the relationship between it and the vascular resistance of each systemic organ.

▶ Defines vascular compliance and states how the volume–pressure curves for arteries and veins differ.

▶ Predicts what will happen to venous volume when venous smooth muscle contracts or when venous transmural pressure increases.

▶ Describes the role of arterial compliance in storing energy for blood circulation.

▶ Describes the auscultation technique for determining arterial systolic and diastolic pressures.

▶ Identifies the physical bases of the Korotkoff sounds.

▶ Indicates the relationship between arterial pressure, cardiac output, and total peripheral resistance and predicts how arterial pressure will be altered when cardiac output and/or total peripheral resistance changes.

▶ Given arterial systolic and diastolic pressures, estimates mean arterial pressure.

▶ Indicates the relationship between pulse pressure, stroke volume, and arterial compliance and predicts how pulse pressure will be changed by changes in stroke volume, or arterial compliance.

▶ Describes how arterial compliance changes with age and how this affects arterial pulse pressure.

Recall from Chapter 1 that the primary job of the cardiovascular system is to maintain "homeostasis" within a body that contains billions of closely spaced individual cells. Homeostasis implies that each and every cell in the body is continually bathed in a local environment of constant composition that is optimal for cell function. In essence, the peripheral vascular system is a sophisticated irrigation system. Blood flow is continually delivering nutrients to and removing waste products from the local interstitial environment throughout the body each and every minute, as required.

The heart supplies the pumping power required to create flow through the system. Because of the heart's action, pressure at the inlet (the aorta) of the vascular network is higher than that at its outlets (the vena cavae). Everywhere within the vascular system, blood always flows passively "downhill" from higher pressure to lower pressure according to well-known physical rules. Like water flowing downhill, blood seeks to travel along the path of least resistance. Consequently, the peripheral vascular system changes the resistance of its various pathways to direct blood flow to where it is needed.

To appreciate the elegant design of our peripheral vascular system, it is essential to understand the physical constraints within which it must operate. This chapter begins with a description of the mechanisms responsible for the transport of dissolved substances through the vascular system and the movement of these substances and fluid from capillaries to and from the interstitial space. Next, the basic equation for flow through a single vessel ($\dot{Q} = \Delta P/R$, presented in Chapter 1) is applied to the complex network of branching vessels that actually exist in the cardiovascular system. Then, the consequences of the elastic (balloon-like) properties of the large-diameter arteries and veins on overall cardiovascular system operation are considered. Finally, the principles behind the routine clinical measurement of arterial blood pressure are presented along with the conclusions about overall cardiovascular function that can be made from the information.

CARDIOVASCULAR TRANSPORT

The Fick Principle

 Substances are carried between organs within the cardiovascular system by the process of *convective transport,* the simple process of being swept along with the flow of the blood in which they are contained. The rate at which a substance (X) is transported by this process depends solely on the concentration of the substance in the blood and the blood flow rate.

$$\text{Transport rate} = \text{flow rate} \times \text{concentration}$$

or

$$\dot{X} = \dot{Q}[X]$$

where $\dot{X}$ = rate of transport of X (mass/time)
$\dot{Q}$ = blood flow rate (volume/time)
$[X]$ = concentration of X in blood (mass/volume)

It is evident from the preceding equation that only two methods are available for altering the rate at which a substance is carried to an organ: (1) a change in the blood flow rate through the organ or (2) a change in the arterial blood concentration of the substance. The preceding equation might be used, for example, to calculate how much oxygen is carried to a certain skeletal muscle each minute. Note, however, that this calculation would not indicate whether the muscle actually used the oxygen carried to it.

One can extend the convective transport principle to determine a tissue's rate of utilization (or production) of a substance by simultaneously considering the transport rate of the substance to *and from* the tissue. The relationship that results is referred to as the *Fick principle* (Adolf Fick, a German physician, 1829–1901) and may be formally stated as follows:

$$\dot{X}_{tc} = \dot{Q}([X]_a - [X]_v)$$

where $\dot{X}_{tc}$ = transcapillary efflux rate of X (mass/time)
$\dot{Q}$ = blood flow rate (volume/time)
$[X]_{a,v}$ = arterial and venous concentrations of X

The Fick principle essentially says that the amount of a substance that goes into an organ in a given period ($\dot{Q}[X]_a$) minus the amount that comes out ($\dot{Q}[X]_v$) must equal the tissue utilization rate of that substance. (If the tissue is producing substance X, then the above equation will yield a negative utilization rate.)

Recall that one method for determining cardiac output described in Chapter 3 used the Fick principle to calculate the blood flow rate through the systemic circulation. In that case, the known variables included the systemic tissue oxygen consumption rate and the concentrations of oxygen in arterial blood and mixed venous blood, and the above equation was rearranged to solve for the blood flow rate ($\dot{Q}$).

Transcapillary Solute Diffusion

Capillaries act as efficient exchange sites where most substances cross the capillary walls simply by *passively diffusing* from regions of high concentration to regions of low concentration.[1] As in any diffusion situation, there are four factors that determine the diffusion rate of a substance between the blood and the interstitial fluid: (1) the concentration difference, (2) the surface area for exchange, (3) the diffusion distance, and (4) the permeability of the capillary wall to the diffusing substance.[2]

Capillary beds allow huge amounts of materials to enter and leave blood because they maximize the area across which exchange can occur while minimizing the distance over which the diffusing substances must travel. Capillaries are extremely fine vessels with a *lumen* (inside) diameter of approximately 5 μm, a wall thickness of approximately 1 μm, and an average length of perhaps 0.5 mm. (For comparison, a human hair is roughly 100 μm in diameter.) Capillaries are distributed in incredible numbers in organs and communicate intimately with all regions of the interstitial space. It is estimated that there are approximately 10^{10} capillaries in the systemic organs with a collective surface area of approximately 100 m^2. That is roughly the area of one player's side of a single tennis court. Recall from Chapter 1 that no cell is more than approximately 10 μm (less than 1/10th the thickness of paper) from a capillary. Diffusion is a tremendously powerful mechanism for material exchange when operating over such a short distance and through such a large area. We are far from being able to duplicate—in an artificial lung or kidney, for example—the favorable geometry for diffusional exchange that exists in our own tissues.

As illustrated in Figure 6–1, the capillary wall itself consists of only a single thickness of endothelial cells joined to form a tube. The ease with which a particular solute crosses the capillary wall is expressed in a parameter called its capillary *permeability*. Permeability takes into account all the factors (diffusion coefficient, diffusion distance, and surface area)—except concentration difference—that affect the rate at which a solute crosses the capillary wall.

Careful experimental studies on how rapidly different substances cross capillary walls indicate that two fundamentally distinct pathways exist for transcapillary exchange. Lipid-soluble substances, such as the gases—oxygen and carbon dioxide,

---

[1] Evidence indicates that the capillary endothelial cells can metabolize or produce certain substances. In these special cases, the capillary wall cannot be considered as a passive barrier between the intravascular and interstitial compartments.

[2] These factors are combined in an equation (Fick's first law of diffusion), which describes the rate of diffusion ($\dot{X}_d$) of a substance X across a barrier: $\dot{X}_d = DA\ \Delta[X]/\Delta L$, $\Delta P_1 = \dot{Q}R_1$, where D, A, $\Delta[X]$, and ΔL represent the diffusion coefficient, surface area, concentration difference, and diffusion distance, respectively.

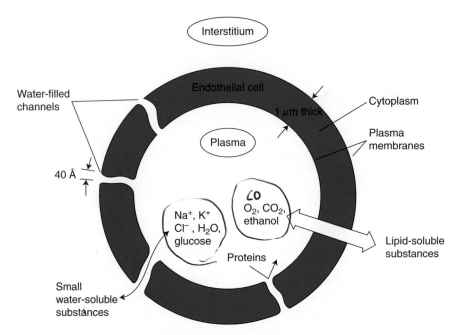

Figure 6–1. Pathways for transcapillary solute diffusion.

cross the capillary wall easily. Because the lipid endothelial cell plasma membranes are not a significant diffusion barrier for lipid-soluble substances, transcapillary movement of these substances can occur through the entire capillary surface area.

The capillary permeability to small polar particles such as sodium and potassium ions is about 10,000-fold less than that for oxygen. Nevertheless, the capillary permeability to small ions is several orders of magnitude higher than the permeability that would be expected if the ions were forced to move through the lipid plasma membranes. It is therefore postulated that capillaries are somehow perforated at intervals with water-filled channels or *pores.*[3] Calculations from diffusion data indicate that the collective cross-sectional area of the pores relative to the total capillary surface area varies greatly between capillaries in different organs. Brain capillaries appear to be very tight (have few pores), whereas capillaries in the kidney and fluid-producing glands are much more leaky. On the average, however, pores constitute only a very small fraction of total capillary surface area—perhaps 0.01%. This area is, nevertheless, sufficient to allow very rapid equilibration of small water-soluble substances between the plasma and interstitial fluids of most organs. Thus, the concentrations of inorganic ions measured in a plasma sample can be taken to indicate their concentrations throughout the entire extracellular space.

---

[3] Pores, as such, are not readily apparent in electron micrographs of capillary endothelial cells. Most believe the pores are really clefts in the junctions between endothelial cells.

An effective maximum diameter of about 40 Å has been assigned to individual pores because substances with molecular diameters larger than this essentially do not cross capillary walls.[4] Thus, albumin and other proteins in the plasma are normally confined to the plasma space.[5]

ENDOTHELIAL CELLS

In addition to forming capillaries, a layer of endothelial cells lines the entire cardiovascular system—including the heart chambers and valves. Because of their ubiquitous and intimate contact with blood, endothelial cells have evolved to serve many functions other than acting as a barrier to transcapillary solute and water exchange. For example, endothelial cell membranes contain specific enzymes that convert some circulating hormones from inactive to active forms. Endothelial cells are also intimately involved in producing substances that lead to blood clot formation and the stemming of bleeding in the event of tissue injury. Moreover, and as discussed in the next chapter, the endothelial cells lining muscular vessels such as arterioles can produce vasoactive substances that act on the smooth muscle cells that surround them to influence arteriolar diameter.

Transcapillary Fluid Movement

In addition to providing a diffusion pathway for polar molecules, the water-filled channels that traverse capillary walls permit fluid flow through the capillary wall. Net shifts of fluid between the capillary and interstitial compartments are important for a host of physiological functions, including the maintenance of circulating blood volume, intestinal fluid absorption, tissue edema formation, and saliva, sweat, and urine production. Net fluid movement out of capillaries is referred to as *filtration*, and fluid movement into capillaries is called *reabsorption.*

Fluid flows through transcapillary channels in response to pressure differences between the interstitial and intracapillary fluids according to the basic flow equation. However, both *hydrostatic* and *osmotic pressures* influence transcapillary fluid movement. How hydrostatic pressure provides the driving force for causing blood flow along vessels has been discussed previously. The hydrostatic pressure inside capillaries, P_c, is about 25 mmHg and is the driving force that causes blood to return to the right side of the heart from the capillaries of systemic organs. In addition, however, the 25-mmHg hydrostatic intracapillary pressure tends to cause fluid to flow through the transcapillary pores into the interstitium where the hydrostatic pressure (P_i) is near 0 mmHg. Thus, there is normally a large hydrostatic pressure difference favoring fluid filtration across the capillary wall. Our entire plasma volume would

---

[4] The precise mechanism responsible for this size selectivity remains controversial. It may stem from the actual physical dimensions of the "pores," or it may represent the filtering properties of a fiber matrix that either covers or fills the pores.

[5] In reality, macromolecules do cross capillary walls ever so slowly by a pinocytotic mechanism sometimes referred to as the "large pore" system. Even with this special system, the capillary protein permeability is still about 1000-fold less than either sodium or glucose permeability.

soon be in the interstitium if there were not some counteracting force tending to draw fluid into the capillaries. The balancing force is an osmotic pressure that arises from the fact that plasma has a higher protein concentration than does interstitial fluid.

Recall that water always tends to move from regions of low to regions of high total solute concentration in establishing osmotic equilibrium. Also, recall that osmotic forces are quantitatively expressed in terms of osmotic pressure. The osmotic pressure of a given solution is defined as the hydrostatic pressure necessary to prevent osmotic water movement into the test solution when it is exposed to pure water across a membrane permeable only to water. The total osmotic pressure of a solution is proportional to the total number of solute particles in the solution. Plasma, for example, has a total osmotic pressure of approximately 5000 mmHg—nearly all of which is attributable to dissolved mineral salts such as NaCl and KCl. As discussed, the capillary permeability to small ions is quite high. Their concentrations in plasma and interstitial fluid are very nearly equal and, consequently, they do not affect transcapillary fluid movement.

There is however a small but important difference in the osmotic pressures of plasma and interstitial fluid that is due to the presence of albumin and other proteins in the plasma, which are normally absent from the interstitial fluid. A special term, *oncotic pressure*, is used to denote the portion of a solution's total osmotic pressure that is due to particles that do not move freely across capillaries.[6] Because of the plasma proteins, the oncotic pressure of plasma (π_c) is approximately 25 mmHg. Because of the absence of proteins, the oncotic pressure of the interstitial fluid (π_i) is near 0 mmHg. Thus, there is normally a large osmotic force for fluid reabsorption into capillaries. The forces that influence transcapillary fluid movement are summarized in the left side of Figure 6–2.

The relationship among the factors that influence transcapillary fluid movement, known as the *Starling hypothesis*,[7] can be expressed by the equation:

$$\text{Net filtration rate} = K[(P_c - P_i) - (\pi_c - \pi_i)]$$

where P_c = the hydrostatic pressure of intracapillary fluid
$\quad\pi_c$ = the oncotic pressure of intracapillary fluid
P_i and π_i = the same quantities for interstitial fluid
$\quad K$ = a constant expressing how readily fluid can move across capillaries (essentially the reciprocal of the resistance to fluid flow through the capillary wall)

Fluid balance within a tissue (the absence of net transcapillary water movement) occurs when the bracketed term in this equation is zero. This equilibrium may be upset by alterations in any of the four pressure terms. The pressure imbalances

---

[6] This osmotic force is also called "colloid osmotic pressure."
[7] After the British physiologist Ernest Starling (1866–1927).

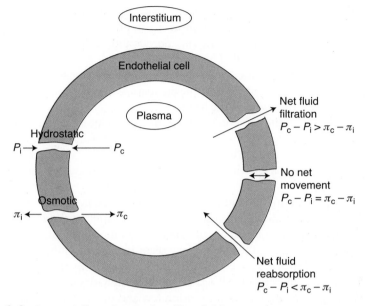

Figure 6–2. Factors influencing transcapillary fluid movement.

that cause capillary filtration and reabsorption are indicated in the right side of Figure 6–2.

In most tissues, rapid net filtration of fluid is abnormal and causes tissue swelling as a result of excess fluid in the interstitial space (edema). For example, a substance called *histamine* is often released in damaged tissue. One of the actions of histamine is to increase capillary permeability to the extent that proteins leak into the interstitium. Net filtration and edema accompany histamine release, in part, because the oncotic pressure difference ($\pi_c - \pi_i$) is reduced below normal.

Transcapillary fluid filtration is not always detrimental. Indeed, fluid-producing organs such as salivary glands and kidneys utilize high intracapillary hydrostatic pressure to produce continual net filtration. Moreover, in certain abnormal situations, such as severe loss of blood volume through hemorrhage, the net fluid reabsorption accompanying diminished intracapillary hydrostatic pressure helps restore the volume of circulating fluid.

Lymphatic System

Despite the extremely low capillary permeability to proteins, these molecules as well as other large particles such as long-chain fatty acids and bacteria find their way into the interstitial space. If such particles are allowed to accumulate in the interstitial space, filtration forces will ultimately exceed reabsorption forces and edema will result. The lymphatic system represents a pathway by which large molecules reenter the circulating blood.

⚡(4) The lymphatic system begins in the tissues with blind-end lymphatic capillaries that are roughly equivalent in size to but less numerous than regular capillaries. These capillaries are very porous and easily collect large particles accompanied by interstitial fluid. This fluid, called *lymph*, moves through the converging lymphatic vessels, is filtered through lymph nodes where bacteria and particulate matter are removed, and reenters the circulatory system near the point where the blood enters the right side of the heart.

Flow of lymph from the tissues toward the entry point into the circulatory system is promoted by two factors: (1) increases in tissue interstitial pressure (due to fluid accumulation or to movement of surrounding tissue) and (2) contractions of the lymphatic vessels themselves. Valves located in these vessels also prevent backward flow.

Roughly 2.5 L of lymphatic fluid enters the cardiovascular system each day. In the steady state, this indicates a total body *net* transcapillary fluid filtration rate of 2.5 L per day. When compared with the total amount of blood that circulates each day (approximately 7000 L), this may seem like an insignificant amount of net capillary fluid leakage. However, lymphatic blockage is a very serious problem and is accompanied by severe swelling. Thus, the lymphatics play a critical role in keeping the interstitial protein concentration low and in removing excess capillary filtrate from the tissues.

BASIC VASCULAR FUNCTION

Resistance and Flow in Networks of Vessels

In Chapter 1, it was asserted that the basic flow equation ($\dot{Q} = \Delta P/R$) may be applied to networks of tubes as well as to individual tubes. The reason is that any network of resistances, however complex, can always be reduced to a single "equivalent" resistor that relates the total flow through the network to the pressure difference across the network. Of course, one way of finding the overall resistance of a network is to perform an experiment to see how much flow goes through it for a given pressure difference between its inlet and outlet. Another approach to finding the overall resistance of a network is to calculate it from knowledge of the resistances of the individual elements in the network and how they are connected. To do so, one needs to apply the parallel and series resistance formulas presented below. These formulas may look familiar because they are analogous to those by which networks of electrical resistances are analyzed with Ohm's law ($I = V/R$).

When vessels with individual resistances $R_1, R_2, \ldots, R_n$ are connected in series, the overall resistance of the network is given by the following formula:

$$R_s = R_1 + R_2 + \cdots + R_n$$

Figure 6–3A shows an example of three vessels connected *in series* between some region where the pressure is P_i and another region with a lower pressure P_o, so that the total pressure difference across the network, ΔP, is equal to $P_i - P_o$. By the

Figure 6–3. Series resistance network.

series resistance equation, the total resistance across this network (R_s) is equal to $R_1 + R_2 + R_3$. By the basic flow equation, the flow through the network ($\dot{Q}$) is equal to $\Delta P/R_s$. It should be intuitively obvious that $\dot{Q}$ is the flow (volume/time) through each of the elements in the series as indicated in Figure 6–3B. (Fluid particles may move with different velocities, distance/time, in different elements of a series network, but the volume that passes through each element in a minute must be identical.)

As shown in Figure 6–3C, a portion of the total pressure drop across the network occurs within each element of the series. The pressure drop across any element in the series can be calculated by applying the basic flow equation to that element, for example, $\Delta P_1 = \dot{Q}R_1$. Note that the largest portion of the overall pressure drop will occur across the element in the series with the largest resistance to flow (R_2 in Figure 6–3).

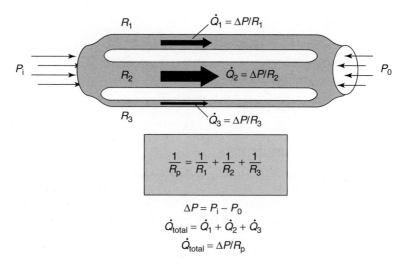

$$\Delta P = P_i - P_0$$
$$\dot{Q}_{total} = \dot{Q}_1 + \dot{Q}_2 + \dot{Q}_3$$
$$\dot{Q}_{total} = \Delta P/R_p$$

Figure 6–4. Parallel resistance network.

As indicated in Figure 6–4, when several tubes with individual resistances R_1, $R_2, \ldots, R_n$ are brought together to form a *parallel* network of vessels, one can calculate a single overall resistance for the parallel network R_p according to the following formula:

$$\frac{1}{R_p} = \frac{1}{R_1} + \frac{1}{R_2} + \cdots + \frac{1}{R_n}$$

The total flow through a parallel network is determined by $\Delta P/R_p$. As the preceding equation implies, the overall resistance of any parallel network will always be less than that of any of the elements in the network. (In the special case where the individual elements that form the network have identical resistances R_x, the overall resistance of the network is equal to the resistance of an individual element divided by the number of n of parallel elements in the network: $R_p = R_x/n$.) In general, the more parallel elements that occur in the network, the lower the overall resistance of the network. Thus, for example, a capillary bed that consists of many individual capillary vessels in parallel can have a very low overall resistance to flow even though the resistance of a single capillary is relatively high.

As indicated in Figure 6–4, the basic flow equation may be applied to any single element in the network or to the network as a whole. For example, the flow through only the first element of the network ($\dot{Q}_1$) is given by $\dot{Q}_1 = \Delta P/R_1$, whereas the flow through the entire parallel network is given by $\dot{Q}_p = \Delta P/R_p$.

The series and parallel resistance equations may be used alternately to analyze resistance networks of great complexity. For example, any or all the series resistances shown in Figure 6–3 could actually represent the calculated overall resistance of many vessels arranged in parallel.

Peripheral Blood Flow Velocities

It is important to make the distinction between blood flow (volume/time) and blood flow velocity (distance/time) in the peripheral vascular system. Consider the analogy of a stream whose water moves with greater velocity through shallow rapids than it does through an adjacent deep pool. The volume of water passing through the pool in a day (volume/time = flow), however, must equal that passing through the rapids in the same day. In such a series arrangement, the flow is the same at all points along the channel but the flow velocity varies inversely with the local cross-sectional area. The situation is the same in the peripheral vasculature, where blood flows most rapidly in the region with the smallest total cross-sectional area (the aorta) and most slowly in the region with the largest total cross-sectional area (the capillary beds). Regardless of the differences in velocity, when the cardiac output (flow into the aorta) is 5 L/min, the flow through the systemic capillaries (or arterioles, or venules) is also 5 L/min. The changes in flow velocity that occur as blood passes through the peripheral vascular system are shown in the top trace in Figure 6–5. These are a

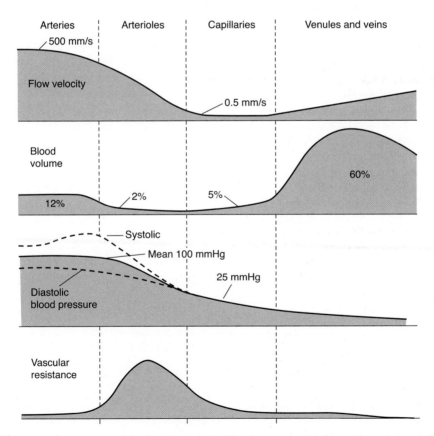

Figure 6–5. Flow velocities, blood volumes, blood pressures, and vascular resistances in the peripheral vasculature from aorta to right atrium.

Figure 6–6. Laminar and turbulent flow patterns.

direct consequence of the variations in total cross-sectional area that were indicated in Figure 1–8.

 The important consequence of this slow flow through the capillaries is that it allows sufficient time for adequate solute and fluid exchange between the vascular and interstitial compartments.

Blood normally flows through all vessels in the cardiovascular system in an orderly streamlined manner called *laminar flow*. With laminar flow, there is a parabolic velocity profile across the tube as shown in the left side of Figure 6–6. Velocity is fastest along the central axis of the tube and falls to zero at the wall. The concentric layers of fluid with different velocities slip smoothly over one another. Little mixing occurs between fluid layers so that individual particles move in straight streamlines parallel to the axis of the flow. Laminar flow is very efficient because little energy is wasted on anything but producing forward fluid motion.

Because blood is a viscous fluid, its movement through a vessel exerts a *shear stress* on the walls of the vessel. This is a force that wants to drag the inside surface (the endothelial cell layer) of the vessel along with the flow. With laminar flow, the shear stress on the wall of a vessel is proportional to the rate of flow through it.[8] The endothelial cells that line a vessel are able to sense (and possibly respond to) changes in the rate of blood flow through the vessel by detecting changes in the shear stress on them. Shear stress may also be an important factor in certain pathological situations. For example, atherosclerotic plaques tend to form preferentially near branches off large arteries where, for complex hemodynamic reasons beyond the scope of this text, high shear stresses exist.

When blood is forced to move with too high a velocity through a narrow opening, the normal laminar flow pattern may break down into the *turbulent flow* pattern shown in the right side of Figure 6–6.[9] With turbulent flow, there is much internal mixing and friction. When the flow within a vessel is turbulent, the vessel's resistance to flow is significantly higher than that predicted from the Poiseuille equation given in Chapter 1. Turbulent flow also generates sound,

---

[8] With pure laminar flow of a homogeneous fluid in a uniform smooth round tube, the shear stress (force/surface area σ_s) on the wall is a function of fluid viscosity (η), flow (volume/time, $\dot{Q}$), and the inside radius of the tube (r_i) as follows: $\sigma_s = 4\eta \dot{Q}/\pi r_i^3$.

[9] Turbulence occurs when a parameter called the *Reynolds number* (R_e) exceeds a value of 2000. $R_e = 4\rho \dot{Q}/\pi \eta d_i$, where ρ = fluid density, $\dot{Q}$ = flow (volume/time), η = fluid viscosity, and d_i = inside diameter.

⑤ which can be heard with the aid of a stethoscope. Cardiac murmurs, for example, are manifestations of turbulent flow patterns generated by cardiac valve abnormalities. Detection of sounds from peripheral arteries (bruits) is abnormal and usually indicates significant pathological reduction of a large vessel's cross-sectional area.

Peripheral Blood Volumes

The second trace in Figure 6–5 shows the approximate percentage of the total circulating blood volume that is contained in the different vascular regions of the systemic organs at any instant of time. (Approximately 20% of the total volume is contained in the pulmonary system and the heart chambers and is not accounted for in this figure.)

⑦ Note that most of the circulating blood is contained within the veins of the systemic organs. This diffuse but large blood reservoir is often referred to as the *peripheral venous pool.* A second but smaller reservoir of venous blood, called the *central venous pool,* is contained in the great veins of the thorax and the right atrium. When peripheral veins constrict, blood is displaced from the peripheral venous pool and enters the central pool. An increase in the central venous volume, and thus pressure, enhances cardiac filling, which in turn augments stroke volume according to the Frank–Starling law of the heart. This is an extremely important mechanism of cardiovascular regulation and is discussed in greater detail in Chapter 8.

Peripheral Blood Pressures

Blood pressure decreases in the consecutive segments with the pattern shown in the third trace in Figure 6–5. Recall from Figure 3–1 that aortic pressure fluctuates between a systolic value and a diastolic value with each heartbeat, and the same is true throughout the arterial system. (For complex hemodynamic reasons, the difference between systolic and diastolic pressures actually increases with the distance from the heart in the large arteries.[10]) The average pressure in the arch of the aorta, however, is about 100 mmHg, and this *mean arterial pressure* falls by only a small amount within the arterial system.

A large pressure drop occurs in the arterioles, where the pulsatile nature of the pressure also nearly disappears. The average capillary pressure is approximately 25 mmHg. Pressure continues to decrease in the venules and veins as blood

---

[10] A rigorous analysis of the dynamics of pulsatile fluid flow in tapered, branching, elastic tubes is required to explain such behavior. Pressure does not increase simultaneously throughout the arterial system with the onset of cardiac ejection. Rather, the pressure increase begins at the root of the aorta and travels outward from there. When this rapidly moving pressure wave encounters obstacles such as vessel bifurcations, reflected waves are generated, which travel back toward the heart. These reflected waves can summate with and reinforce the oncoming wave in a manner somewhat analogous to the progressive cresting of surface waves as they impinge on a beach.

returns to the right heart. The central venous pressure (which is the filling pressure for the right side of the heart) is normally very close to 0 mmHg.

Peripheral Vascular Resistances

The bottom trace in Figure 6–5 indicates the relative resistance to flow that exists in each of the consecutive vascular regions. Recall from Chapter 1 that resistance, pressure difference, and flow are related by the basic flow equation $\dot{Q} = \Delta P/R$. Because the flow ($\dot{Q}$) must be the same through each of the consecutive regions indicated in Figure 6–5, the pressure drop that occurs across each of these regions is a direct reflection of the resistance to flow within that region (see Figure 6–3). Thus, the large pressure drop occurring as blood moves through arterioles indicates that arterioles present a large resistance to flow. The mean pressure drops little in arteries because they have little resistance to flow. Similarly, the modest pressure drop that exists across capillaries is a reflection of the fact that the capillary bed has a modest resistance to flow when compared with that of the arteriolar bed. (Recall from Figure 6–4 that the capillary bed can have a low resistance to flow because it is a parallel network of a very large number of individual capillaries.)

Blood flow through many individual organs can vary over a 10-fold or greater range. Because mean arterial pressure is a relatively stable cardiovascular variable, large changes in an organ's blood flow are achieved by changes in its overall vascular resistance to blood flow. The consecutive vascular segments are arranged in series within an organ, and the overall vascular resistance of the organ must equal the sum of the resistances of its consecutive vascular segments:

$$R_{\text{organ}} = R_{\text{arteries}} + R_{\text{arterioles}} + R_{\text{capillaries}} + R_{\text{venules}} + R_{\text{veins}}$$

Because arterioles have such a large vascular resistance in comparison to the other vascular segments, the overall vascular resistance of any organ is determined to a very large extent by the resistance of its arterioles. Arteriolar resistance is, of course, strongly influenced by arteriolar radius (R is proportional to $1/r^4$). Thus, the blood flow through an organ is primarily regulated by adjustments in the internal diameter of arterioles caused by contraction or relaxation of their muscular arteriolar walls.

When the arterioles of an organ change diameter, not only does the flow to the organ change but the manner in which the pressures drop within the organ is also modified. The effects of arteriolar dilation and constriction on the pressure profile within a vascular bed are illustrated in Figure 6–7. Arteriolar constriction causes a greater pressure drop across the arterioles, and this tends to increase the arterial pressure while it decreases the pressure in capillaries and veins. (The arterioles function somewhat like a dam; closing a dam's gates decreases the flow while increasing the level of the reservoir behind it and decreasing the level of its outflow stream.) Conversely, increased organ blood flow caused by arteriolar dilation is accompanied by decreased arterial pressure and increased capillary pressure. Because of the changes in capillary hydrostatic pressure, arteriolar constriction

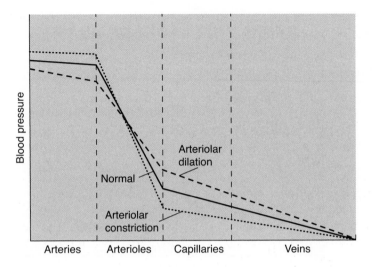

Figure 6–7. Effect of changes in arteriolar resistance on vascular pressures.

tends to cause transcapillary fluid reabsorption whereas arteriolar dilation tends to promote transcapillary fluid filtration.

Total Peripheral Resistance

The overall resistance to flow through the entire systemic circulation is called the *total peripheral resistance*. Because the systemic organs are generally arranged in parallel (Figure 1–2), the vascular resistance of each organ contributes to the total peripheral resistance according to the following parallel resistance equation:

$$\frac{1}{\text{TPR}} = \frac{1}{R_{\text{organ}_1}} + \frac{1}{R_{\text{organ}_2}} + \cdots + \frac{1}{R_{\text{organ}_n}}$$

As discussed later in this chapter, the total peripheral resistance is an important determinant of arterial blood pressure.

Elastic Properties of Arteries and Veins

As indicated earlier, arteries and veins contribute only a small portion to the overall resistance to flow through a vascular bed. Therefore, changes in their diameters have no significant effect on the blood flow through systemic organs. The elastic behavior of arteries and veins is however very important to overall cardiovascular function because they can act as reservoirs and substantial amounts of blood can be stored in them. Arteries or veins behave more like balloons with one pressure throughout rather than as resistive pipes with a flow-related pressure difference from end to end. Thus, think of an "arterial compartment" and a "venous compartment," each with

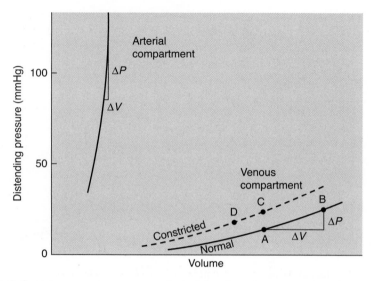

Figure 6–8. Volume–pressure curves of arterial and venous compartments.

an internal pressure that is related to the volume of blood within it at any instant and how elastic (stretchy) its walls are.

The elastic nature of a vascular region is characterized by a parameter called *compliance* (*C*) that describes how much its volume changes (ΔV) in response to a given change in distending pressure (ΔP): $C = \Delta V / \Delta P$. Distending pressure is the difference between the internal and external pressures on the vascular walls.

The volume–pressure curves for the systemic arterial and venous compartments are shown in Figure 6–8. It is immediately apparent from the disparate slopes of the curves in this figure that the elastic properties of arteries and veins are very different. For the arterial compartment, the $\Delta V / \Delta P$ measured near a normal operating pressure of 100 mmHg indicates a compliance of about 2 mL/mmHg. By contrast, the venous pool has a compliance of over 100 mL/mmHg near its normal operating pressure of 5 to 10 mmHg.

Because veins are so compliant, even small changes in peripheral venous pressure can cause a significant amount of the circulating blood volume to shift into or out of the peripheral venous pool. Standing upright, for example, increases venous pressure in the lower extremities and promotes blood accumulation (pooling) in these vessels as might be represented by a shift from point A to point B in Figure 6–8. Fortunately, this process can be counteracted by active venous constriction. The dashed line in Figure 6–8 shows the venous volume–pressure relationship that exists when veins are constricted by activation of venous smooth muscle. In constricted veins, volume may be normal (point C) or even below normal (point D) despite higher than normal venous pressure. Peripheral venous constriction tends to increase peripheral venous pressure and shift blood out of the peripheral venous compartment.

The elasticity of arteries allows them to act as a reservoir on a beat-to-beat basis. Arteries play an important role in converting the pulsatile flow output of the heart into a steady flow through the vascular beds of systemic organs. During the early rapid phase of cardiac ejection, the arterial volume increases because blood is entering the aorta more rapidly than it is passing into systemic arterioles. Thus, part of the work the heart does in ejecting blood goes to stretching the elastic walls of arteries. Toward the end of systole and throughout diastole, arterial volume decreases because the flow out of arteries exceeds flow into the aorta. Previously stretched arterial walls recoil to shorter lengths and in the process give up their stored potential energy. This reconverted energy is what actually does the work of propelling blood through the peripheral vascular beds during diastole. If the arteries were rigid tubes that could not store energy by expanding elastically, arterial pressure would fall immediately to zero with the termination of each cardiac ejection.

MEASUREMENT OF ARTERIAL PRESSURE

Recall that the systemic arterial pressure fluctuates with each heart cycle between a diastolic value (P_D) and a higher systolic value (P_S). Obtaining estimates of an individual's systolic and diastolic pressures is one of the most routine diagnostic techniques available to the physician. The basic principles of the *auscultation* technique used to measure blood pressure are described here with the aid of Figure 6–9.

An inflatable cuff is wrapped around the upper arm, and a device, such as a mercury manometer, is attached to monitor the pressure within the cuff. The cuff is initially inflated with air to a pressure ($\simeq$175 to 200 mmHg) that is well above

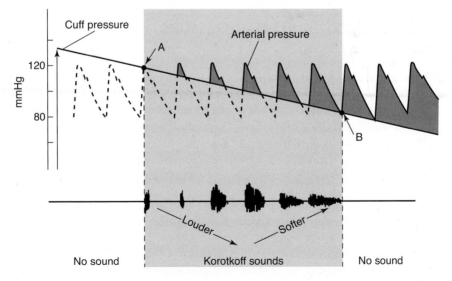

Figure 6–9. Blood pressure measurement by auscultation. Point **A** indicates systolic pressure and point **B** indicates diastolic pressure.

normal systolic values. This pressure is transmitted from the flexible cuff into the upper arm tissues, where it causes all blood vessels to collapse. No blood flows into (or out of) the forearm as long as the cuff pressure is higher than the systolic arterial pressure. After the initial inflation, air is allowed to gradually "bleed" from the cuff so that the pressure within it falls slowly and steadily through the range of arterial pressure fluctuations. The moment the cuff pressure falls below the peak systolic arterial pressure, some blood is able to pass through the arteries beneath the cuff during the systolic phase of the cycle. This flow is intermittent and occurs only over a brief period of each heart cycle. Moreover, because it occurs through partially collapsed vessels beneath the cuff, the flow is turbulent rather than laminar. The intermittent periods of flow beneath the cuff produce tapping sounds, which can be detected with a stethoscope placed over the radial artery at the elbow. As indicated in Figure 6–9, sounds of varying character, known collectively as *Korotkoff sounds*, are heard whenever the cuff pressure is between the systolic and diastolic aortic pressures.

Because there is no blood flow and thus no sound when cuff pressure is higher than systolic arterial pressure, *the highest cuff pressure at which tapping sounds are heard is taken as the systolic arterial pressure.* When the cuff pressure falls below the diastolic pressure, blood flows through the vessels beneath the cuff without periodic interruption and again no sound is detected over the radial artery. *The cuff pressure at which the sounds become muffled or disappear is taken as the diastolic arterial pressure.* The Korotkoff sounds are more distinct when the cuff pressure is near the systolic arterial pressure than when it is near the diastolic pressure. Thus, consistency in determining diastolic pressure by auscultation requires concentration and experience.

DETERMINANTS OF ARTERIAL PRESSURE

Mean Arterial Pressure

 Mean arterial pressure is a critically important cardiovascular variable because it is the average effective pressure that drives blood through the systemic organs. One of the most fundamental equations of cardiovascular physiology is that which indicates how mean arterial pressure ($\bar{P}_A$) is related to cardiac output (CO) and total peripheral resistance (TPR):

$$\bar{P}_A = CO \times TPR$$

This equation is simply a rearrangement of the basic flow equation ($\dot{Q} = \Delta P/R$) applied to the entire systemic circulation with the single assumption that central venous pressure is approximately zero so that $\Delta P = \bar{P}_A$. Note that mean arterial pressure is influenced both by the heart (via cardiac output) and by the peripheral vasculature (via total peripheral resistance). *All changes in mean arterial pressure result from changes in either cardiac output or total peripheral resistance.*

Calculating the true value of mean arterial pressure requires mathematically averaging the arterial pressure waveform over one or more complete heart cycles. Most often, however, we know from auscultation only the systolic and diastolic pressures, yet wish to make some estimate of the mean arterial pressure. Mean arterial pressure necessarily falls between the systolic and diastolic pressures. A useful rule of thumb is that mean arterial pressure ($\bar{P}_A$) is approximately equal to diastolic pressure (P_D) plus one-third of the difference between systolic and diastolic pressures ($P_S - P_D$):

$$\bar{P}_A \simeq P_D + \frac{1}{3}(P_S - P_D)$$

Arterial Pulse Pressure

The *arterial pulse pressure* (P_p) is defined simply as systolic pressure minus diastolic pressure:

$$P_p = P_S - P_D$$

To be able to use pulse pressure to deduce something about how the cardiovascular system is operating, one must do more than just define it. It is important to understand what *determines* pulse pressure; that is, what causes it to be what it is and what can cause it to change. In a previous section of this chapter, there was a brief discussion about how, as a consequence of the compliance of the arterial vessels, arterial pressure increases as arterial blood volume is expanded during cardiac ejection. The magnitude of the pressure increase (ΔP) caused by an increase in arterial volume depends on how large the volume change (ΔV) is and on how compliant (C_A) the arterial compartment is: $\Delta P = \Delta V / C_A$. If, for the moment, the fact that some blood leaves the arterial compartment *during* cardiac ejection is neglected, then the increase in arterial volume during each heartbeat is equal to the stroke volume (SV).

 Thus, pulse pressure is, to a first approximation, equal to stroke volume divided by arterial compliance:

$$P_p \simeq \frac{SV}{C_A}$$

Arterial pulse pressure is approximately 40 mmHg in a normal resting young adult because stroke volume is approximately 80 mL and arterial compliance is approximately 2 mL/mmHg. Pulse pressure tends to increase with age in adults because of a decrease in arterial compliance ("hardening of the arteries"). Arterial volume–pressure curves for a 20-year-old and a 70-year-old are shown in Figure 6–10. The decrease in arterial compliance with age is indicated by the steeper curve for the 70-year-old (more ΔP for a given ΔV) than for the 20-year-old. Thus, a 70-year-old will necessarily have a larger pulse pressure for a given stroke volume than a 20-year-old. As indicated in Figure 6–10, the decrease in arterial compliance

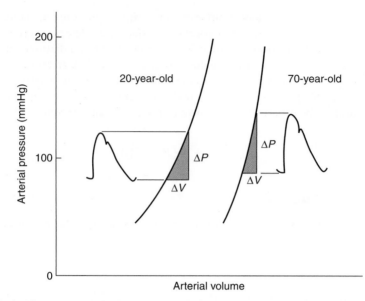

Figure 6–10. Observed effects of aging on the pressure-volume relationship of arteries. Also indicated are normal age-related changes in stroke volume (ΔV) and arterial pressures.

is sufficient to cause increased pulse pressure even though stroke volume tends to decrease with age.

Figure 6–10 also illustrates the fact that arterial blood volume and mean arterial pressure tend to increase with age. The increase in *mean* arterial pressure is *not* caused by the decreased arterial compliance because compliance changes do not directly influence either cardiac output or total peripheral resistance, which are the *sole determinants* of $\bar{P}_A$. Mean arterial pressure tends to increase with age because of an age-dependent increase in total peripheral resistance, which is controlled primarily by arterioles, not arteries.

Arterial compliance also decreases with increasing mean arterial pressure as evidenced by the curvature of the volume–pressure relationships shown in Figure 6–10. Otherwise, arterial compliance is a relatively stable parameter. Thus, most acute changes in arterial pulse pressure are the result of changes in stroke volume.

The preceding equation for pulse pressure is a much-simplified description of some very complex hemodynamic processes. It correctly identifies stroke volume and arterial compliance as the major determinants of arterial pulse pressure but is based on the assumption that no blood leaves the aorta during systolic ejection. Obviously, this is not strictly correct. Furthermore, close examination of Figure 3–1 will reveal that peak systolic pressure is reached even before cardiac ejection is complete. It is therefore not surprising that several factors other than arterial compliance and stroke volume have minor influences on pulse pressure. For example, because the arteries have viscous properties as well as elastic characteristics, faster cardiac ejection caused by increased myocardial contractility tends to increase pulse pressure somewhat even if stroke volume remains constant. Changes in total peripheral resistance, however, have *little or no effect on pulse pressure*, because a change in total peripheral resistance causes parallel changes in both systolic and diastolic pressures.

A common misconception in cardiovascular physiology is that the systolic pressure alone or the diastolic pressure alone indicates the status of a specific cardiovascular variable. For example, high diastolic pressure is often taken to indicate high total peripheral resistance. This is not necessarily so because high diastolic pressure can exist with normal (or even reduced) total peripheral resistance if the heart rate and cardiac output are high. Both systolic and diastolic pressures are influenced by the heart rate, stroke volume, total peripheral resistance, and C_A.[11] The student should not attempt to interpret systolic and diastolic pressure values independently. Interpretation is much more straightforward when the focus is on mean arterial pressure ($\overline{P}_A = CO \times TPR$) and arterial pulse pressure ($P_p \simeq SV/C_A$). (See study question 6–14.)

KEY CONCEPTS

Within the cardiovascular system, convection is used to transport substances between capillary beds and diffusion is used to transport substances between blood and tissue.

Water may move out of (filtration) or into (reabsorption) capillaries depending on the net balance of hydrostatic and osmotic forces across capillary walls.

Plasma proteins are responsible for the major osmotic force across capillary walls.

Lymphatic vessels serve to remove excess filtrate from tissues and keep interstitial protein concentration low.

The velocity of blood flow is inversely proportional to the total cross-sectional area of the vascular segment and is slowest in capillaries.

---

[11] The equations presented in this and preceding chapters can be solved simultaneously to show that

$$P_S \simeq SV \times HR \times TPR + \frac{2}{3}\frac{SV}{C_A}$$

$$P_D \simeq SV \times HR \times TPR - \frac{1}{3}\frac{SV}{C_A}$$

6 Turbulent blood flow is abnormal and makes noise (murmurs and bruits).

 7 Veins contain most of the total blood volume.

 8 Arterioles contribute most to the resistance to flow through organs.

 9 Arteriolar constriction tends to reduce flow through an organ, reduce capillary hydrostatic pressure, and promote transcapillary fluid reabsorption within the organ.

10 Venous constriction is important for cardiac filling and the ability to cope with blood loss.

 11 Because arteries are elastic, the intermittent flow from the heart is converted to continuous flow through capillaries.

 12 Mean systemic arterial pressure is determined by the product of cardiac output and total peripheral resistance.

13 Changes in arterial pulse pressure reflect changes in stroke volume and/or the compliance of the arterial space.

 ## STUDY QUESTIONS

6-1. Determine the rate of glucose uptake by an exercising skeletal muscle ($\dot{G}_m$) from the following data:

Arterial blood glucose concentration, $[G]_a = 50$ mg/100 mL
Muscle venous blood glucose concentration, $[G]_v = 30$ mg/100 mL
Blood flow, $\dot{Q} = 60$ mL/min

3 mg/min

6-2. Determine the direction of transcapillary fluid movement ($\dot{F}$) within a tissue, given the following data:

Capillary hydrostatic pressure, $P_c = 28$ mmHg
Plasma oncotic pressure, $\pi_c = 24$ mmHg
Tissue hydrostatic pressure, $P_i = -4$ mmHg
Tissue oncotic pressure, $\pi_i = 0$ mmHg

filtration
out.

6-3. Which of the following conditions favor edema formation?
a. lymphatic blockage
b. thrombophlebitis (venous clot)

All

    c. decreased plasma protein concentration

    d. greatly increased capillary pore size

6–4. Assume that three vessels with identical dimensions are combined into a network of one vessel followed by a parallel combination of the other two and that a pressure (P_i) is applied to the inlet of the first vessel while a lower pressure (P_o) exists at the outlet of the parallel pair.

    a. Find the overall resistance of the network (R_n) if the resistance of each vessel is equal to R_e.

    b. Is the pressure (P_j) at the central junction of the network closer to P_i or P_o?

    c. Use the basic flow equation to derive an equation that relates the pressure drop across the input vessel ($P_i - P_j$) to the total pressure drop across the network ($P_i - P_o$).

6–5. Given the following data, calculate an individual's total peripheral resistance (TPR):

    Mean arterial pressure, $\bar{P}_A = 100\ mmHg$

    Central venous pressure, $P_{CV} = 0\ mmHg$

    Cardiac output, $CO = 6\ L/min$

6–6. The TPR to blood flow is greater than the resistance to flow through any of the systemic organs. True or false?

6–7. Other factors being equal, a decrease in the renal vascular resistance will increase TPR. True or false?

6–8. Constriction of arterioles in an organ promotes reabsorption of interstitial fluid from that organ. True or false?

6–9. Chronic elevation of arterial pressure requires that either cardiac output or TPR (or both) be chronically elevated. True or false?

6–10. Whenever cardiac output is increased, mean arterial pressure must also be increased. True or false?

6–11. Acute increases in arterial pulse pressure usually result from increases in stroke volume. True or false?

6–12. An increase in TPR increases diastolic pressure (P_D) more than systolic pressure (P_S). True or false?

6–13. Estimate the mean arterial pressure when the measured arterial pressure is 110/70 mmHg.

6–14. At rest the patient has a pulse rate of 70 beats per minute and an arterial blood pressure of 119/80 mmHg. During exercise on a treadmill, pulse rate is 140 beats per minute and blood pressure is 135/90 mmHg. Use this information to estimate the exercise-related changes in the following variables:

    a. stroke volume

    b. cardiac output

    c. total peripheral resistance (TPR)

6–15. Which of the following is consistent with a normal mean arterial pressure but an abnormally high arterial pulse pressure?

    a. low stroke volume

    b. high heart rate

    c. decreased total peripheral resistance

    d. increased arterial stiffness

    e. aortic valve stenosis

6-16. Which of the following substances is likely to move most easily across a skeletal muscle capillary wall?

  a. potassium
  b. glucose
  c. oxygen
  d. water
  e. albumin

6-17. In which of the following vessels do red cells move with the fastest speed (distance/time)?

  a. arteries
  b. arterioles
  c. capillaries
  d. venules
  e. veins

Vascular Control

OBJECTIVES

The student understands the general mechanisms involved in local vascular control:

▶ *Identifies the major ways in which smooth muscle differs anatomically and functionally from striated muscle.*

▶ *Lists the steps leading to cross-bridge cycling in smooth muscle.*

▶ *Lists the major ion channels involved in the regulation of membrane potential in smooth muscle.*

▶ *Describes the processes of electromechanical and pharmacomechanical coupling in smooth muscle.*

▶ *Defines basal tone.*

▶ *Lists several substances potentially involved in local metabolic control.*

▶ *States the local metabolic vasodilator hypothesis.*

▶ *Describes how vascular tone is influenced by prostaglandins, histamine, and bradykinin.*

▶ *Describes the myogenic response of blood vessels.*

▶ *Defines active and reactive hyperemia and indicates a possible mechanism for each.*

▶ *Defines autoregulation of blood flow and briefly describes the metabolic, myogenic, and tissue pressure theories of autoregulation.*

▶ *Defines neurogenic tone and describes how sympathetic (and parasympathetic) neural influences can alter it.*

▶ *Describes how vascular tone is influenced by circulating catecholamines, vasopressin, and angiotensin II.*

▶ *Lists the major influences on venous diameters.*

▶ *Describes, in general, how control of flow differs between organs with strong local metabolic control of arteriolar tone and organs with strong neurogenic control of arteriolar tone.*

The student knows the dominant mechanisms of flow and blood volume control in the major body organs:

▶ *States the relative importance of local metabolic and neural control of coronary blood flow.*

▶ *Defines systolic compression and indicates its relative importance to blood flow in the endocardial and epicardial regions of the right and left ventricular walls.*

▶ *Describes the major mechanisms of flow and blood volume control in each of the following specific systemic organs: skeletal muscle, brain, splanchnic organs, skin, and kidney.*

▶ *States why mean pulmonary arterial pressure is lower than mean systemic arterial pressure.*

▶ *Describes how pulmonary vascular control differs from that in systemic organs.*

 Because the body's metabolic needs are continually changing, the cardiovascular system must continually make adjustments in the diameter of its vessels. The purposes of these vascular changes are (1) to efficiently distribute the cardiac output among tissues with different current needs (the job of arterioles) and (2) to regulate the distribution of blood volume and cardiac filling (the job of veins). In this chapter we discuss our current understanding of how all this is accomplished.

VASCULAR SMOOTH MUSCLE

Vascular diameter adjustments are made by regulating the contractile activity of vascular smooth muscle cells, which are present in the walls of all vessels except capillaries. The task of the vascular smooth muscle is unique, because to maintain a certain vessel diameter in the face of the continual distending pressure of the blood within it, the vascular smooth muscle must be able to sustain active tension for prolonged periods.

There are many functional characteristics that distinguish smooth muscle from either skeletal or cardiac muscle. For example, when compared with these other muscle types, smooth muscle cells:

1. Contract and relax much more slowly.
2. Develop active tension over a greater range of muscle lengths.
3. Can change their contractile activity as a result of action potentials or changes in resting membrane potential.
4. May change their contractile activity in the absence of changes in membrane potential.
5. Maintain tension for prolonged periods at low energy cost.
6. Can be activated by stretch.

Contractile Machinery

Vascular smooth muscle cells are small (approximately 5 μm × 50 μm) spindle-shaped cells usually arranged circumferentially or at small helical angles in blood vessel walls. In many but not all vessels, adjacent smooth muscle cells are electrically connected by gap junctions similar to those found in the myocardium.

Just as in other muscle types, smooth muscle force development and shortening are the result of cross-bridge interaction between thick and thin contractile filaments composed of myosin and actin, respectively. In smooth muscle, however, these filaments are not arranged in regular, repeating sarcomere units. As a consequence, "smooth" muscle cells lack the microscopically visible striations, characteristic of skeletal and cardiac muscle cells. The actin filaments in smooth muscle are much longer than those in striated muscle. Many of these actin filaments attach to the inner surface of the cell at structures called *dense bands*. In the interior of the cell, actin filaments do not attach to Z-lines but rather anchor to small transverse structures called *dense bodies* that are themselves tethered to the surface membrane by cable-like *intermediate filaments*. Myosin filaments are interspersed between the smooth muscle actin filaments but in a more haphazard fashion than the regular interweaving pattern of striated muscle. In striated muscle, the contractile filaments are invariably aligned with the long axis of the cell whereas in smooth muscle, many contractile filaments travel obliquely or even transversely to the long axis of the cell. Despite the absence of organized sarcomeres, changes in smooth muscle length affect its ability to actively develop tension. Perhaps because of the long actin filaments and the lack of sarcomere arrangement, smooth muscle can develop tension over a greater range of length changes than either skeletal or cardiac muscle.

As in striated muscle, the strength of the cross-bridge interaction between thick and thin filaments in smooth muscle is controlled primarily by changes in the intracellular free Ca^{2+} level, which range from approximately 10^{-8} M in the relaxed muscle to 10^{-5} M during maximal contraction. However, the sequence of steps linking an increased free Ca^{2+} level to contractile filament interaction is different in smooth muscle than in striated muscle. In the smooth muscle:

1. Ca^{2+} first forms a complex with the calcium-binding protein *calmodulin*.
2. The Ca^{2+}–calmodulin complex then activates a phosphorylating enzyme called *myosin light-chain kinase*.
3. This enzyme causes phosphorylation by adenosine triphosphate (ATP) of the light-chain protein that is a portion of the cross-bridge head of myosin.
4. Myosin light-chain phosphorylation enables cross-bridge formation and cycling during which energy from ATP is utilized for tension development and shortening.

Smooth muscle is also unique in that once tension is developed, it can be maintained at very low energy costs, that is, without the need to continually split ATP in cross-bridge cycling. The mechanisms responsible are still somewhat unclear but presumably involve very slowly cycling or even noncycling cross-bridges. This is often referred to as the *latch state* and may involve light-chain dephosphorylation of attached cross-bridges. Also by mechanisms that are yet incompletely understood, it is apparent that vascular smooth muscle contractile activity is regulated not only by changes in intracellular free Ca^{2+} levels but also by changes in the Ca^{2+} *sensitivity* of the contractile machinery. Thus, the contractile state of vascular smooth muscle may sometimes change in the absence of changes in intracellular free Ca^{2+} levels.

Membrane Potentials

Smooth muscle cells have resting membrane potentials ranging from -40 to -65 mV and thus are generally lower than those in striated muscle. As in all cells, the resting membrane potential of the smooth muscle is determined largely by the cell permeability to potassium. Many types of K^+ channels have been identified in smooth muscle. The one that seems to be predominantly responsible for determining the resting membrane potential is termed an *inward rectifying-type* K^+ channel. (*Inward rectifying* implies that K^+ ions move into cells through this channel slightly more easily than they move out through it.) There are also *ATP-dependent* K^+ channels that are closed when cellular ATP levels are normal but open if ATP levels fall. Such channels have been proposed to be important in matching organ blood flow to the metabolic state of the tissue.

Smooth muscle cells regularly have action potentials only in certain vessels. When they do occur, smooth muscle action potentials are initiated primarily by inward Ca^{2+} current and are developed slowly like the "slow-type" cardiac action potentials (see Figure 2–2). As in the heart, this inward (depolarizing) Ca^{2+} current flows through a *voltage-operated calcium channel* (VOC); this type of channel is one of several types of calcium channels present in the smooth muscle. The repolarization phase of the action potential occurs primarily by an outward flux of potassium ions through both *delayed* K^+ channels and *calcium-activated* K^+ channels.

Many types of ion channels in addition to those mentioned have been identified in vascular smooth muscle, but in most cases their exact role in cardiovascular function remains obscure. For example, there appear to be nonselective, stretch-sensitive cation channels that may be involved in the response of smooth muscle to stretch. The reader should note, however, that many of the important ion channels in vascular smooth muscle are also important in heart muscle (see Table 2–1).

Electromechanical Versus Pharmacomechanical Coupling

In smooth muscle, changes in intracellular free Ca^{2+} levels can occur both with *and* without changes in membrane potential. The processes involved are called *electromechanical coupling* and *pharmacomechanical coupling*, respectively, and are illustrated in Figure 7–1.

Electromechanical coupling, shown in the left half of Figure 7–1, occurs because the smooth muscle surface membrane contains voltage-operated channels for calcium (the same VOCs that are involved in action potential generation). Membrane depolarization increases the open-state probability of these channels and thus leads to smooth muscle cell contraction and vessel constriction. Conversely, membrane hyperpolarization leads to smooth muscle relaxation and vessel dilation. Because the VOCs for Ca^{2+} are partially activated by the low resting membrane potential of the

Figure 7–1. General mechanisms for activation of the vascular smooth muscle. VOC, voltage-operated Ca^{2+} channel; ROC, receptor-operated Ca^{2+} channel; R, agonist-specific receptor; G, GTP-binding protein; PIP_2, phosphatidylinositol biphosphate; IP_3, inositol triphosphate; DAG, diacylglycerol.

vascular smooth muscle, changes in resting potential can alter the resting calcium influx rate and therefore the basal contractile state.

With pharmacomechanical coupling, chemical agents (eg, released neurotransmitters) can induce smooth muscle contraction without the need for a change in membrane potential. As illustrated in the right side of Figure 7–1, the combination of a vasoconstrictor agonist (such as norepinephrine) with a specific membrane-bound receptor (such as an α_1-adrenergic receptor) initiates events that cause intracellular free Ca^{2+} levels to increase for two reasons. One, the activated receptor may open surface membrane *receptor-operated channels* for Ca^{2+} that allow Ca^{2+} influx from the extracellular fluid. Two, the activated receptor may induce the formation of an intracellular "second messenger," inositol trisphosphate (IP_3), that opens specific channels that release Ca^{2+} from the intracellular sarcoplasmic reticulum stores. In both processes, the activated receptor first stimulates specific guanosine triphosphate-binding proteins (GTP-binding proteins or *G proteins*). Such receptor-associated G proteins seem to represent a general first step through which most membrane receptors operate to initiate their particular cascade of events that ultimately lead to specific cellular responses.

The reader should *not* conclude from Figure 7–1 that all vasoactive chemical agents (chemical agents that cause vascular effects) produce their actions on the smooth muscle without changing membrane potential. In fact, most vasoactive chemical agents do cause changes in membrane potential because their receptors can be linked, by G proteins or other means, to ion channels of many kinds.

Not shown in Figure 7–1 are the processes that remove Ca^{2+} from the cytoplasm of the vascular smooth muscle although they are important as well in determining the free cytosolic Ca^{2+} levels. As in cardiac cells (see Figure 2–7), smooth muscle cells actively pump calcium into the sarcoplasmic reticulum and outward across the sarcolemma. Calcium is also countertransported out of the cell in exchange for sodium.

Mechanisms for Relaxation

Hyperpolarization of the cell membrane is one mechanism for causing smooth muscle relaxation and vessel dilation. In addition, however, there are at least two general mechanisms by which certain chemical vasodilator agents can cause smooth muscle relaxation by pharmacomechanical means. In Figure 7–1, the specific receptor for a chemical vasoconstrictor agent is shown linked by a specific G protein to phospholipase C. In an analogous manner, other specific receptors may be linked by other specific G proteins to other enzymes that produce second messengers other than IP_3. An example is the β_2-adrenergic receptor[1] that is present in arterioles of the skeletal muscle and liver. β_2-Receptors are not innervated but can sometimes be activated by abnormally elevated levels of circulating *epinephrine*. The β_2-receptor is linked by a particular G protein (G_s) to adenylate cyclase. Adenylate cyclase catalyzes the conversion of ATP to cyclic adenosine monophosphate (cAMP). Increased intracellular levels of cAMP cause the activation of protein kinase A, a phosphorylating enzyme that in turn causes phosphorylation of proteins at many sites. The overall result is stimulation of Ca^{2+} efflux, membrane hyperpolarization, and decreased contractile machinery sensitivity to Ca^{2+}—all of which act synergistically to cause vasodilation. In addition to epinephrine, histamine and vasoactive intestinal peptide are vasodilator substances that act through the cAMP pathway.

In addition to cAMP, cyclic guanosine monophosphate (cGMP) is an important intracellular second messenger that causes vascular smooth muscle relaxation by mechanisms that are not yet clear. Nitric oxide is an important vasodilator substance that operates via the cGMP pathway. Nitric oxide can be produced by endothelial cells and also by nitrates, a clinically important class of vasodilator drugs. Nitric oxide is gaseous and easily diffuses into smooth muscle cells, where it activates the enzyme guanylyl cyclase that in turn causes cGMP formation from GTP.

Vascular Tone

Vascular tone is a term commonly used to characterize the general contractile state of a vessel or a vascular region. The "vascular tone" of a region can be taken as an indication of the "level of activation" of the individual smooth muscle cells in that region.

---

[1] Vascular β-receptors are designated β_2-receptors and are pharmacologically distinct from the β_1-receptors found on cardiac cells.

CONTROL OF ARTERIOLAR TONE

As described in Chapter 6, the blood flow through any organ is determined largely by its vascular resistance, which is dependent primarily on the diameter of its arterioles. Consequently, an organ's flow is controlled by factors that influence the arteriolar smooth muscle tone.

Basal Tone

Arterioles remain in a state of partial constriction even when all external influences on them are removed; hence, they are said to have a degree of *basal tone* (sometimes referred to as *intrinsic tone*). The understanding of the mechanism is incomplete, but basal arteriolar tone may be a reflection of the fact that smooth muscle cells inherently and actively resist being stretched as they continually are in pressurized arterioles. Another hypothesis is that the basal tone of arterioles is the result of a tonic production of local vasoconstrictor substances by the endothelial cells that line their inner surface. In any case, this basal tone establishes a baseline of partial arteriolar constriction from which the external influences on arterioles exert their dilating or constricting effects. These influences can be separated into three categories: local influences, neural influences, and hormonal influences.

Local Influences on Arterioles

LOCAL METABOLIC INFLUENCES

The arterioles that control flow through a given organ lie within the organ tissue itself. Thus, arterioles and the smooth muscle in their walls are exposed to the chemical composition of the interstitial fluid of the organ they serve. The interstitial concentrations of many substances reflect the balance between the metabolic activity of the tissue and its blood supply. Interstitial oxygen levels, for example, fall whenever the tissue cells are using oxygen faster than it is being supplied to the tissue by blood flow. Conversely, interstitial oxygen levels rise whenever excess oxygen is being delivered to a tissue from the blood. In nearly all vascular beds, exposure to low oxygen reduces arteriolar tone and causes vasodilation, whereas high oxygen levels cause arteriolar vasoconstriction.[2] Thus, a local feedback mechanism exists that automatically operates on arterioles to regulate a tissue's blood flow in accordance with its metabolic needs. Whenever blood flow and oxygen delivery fall below a tissue's oxygen demands, the oxygen levels around arterioles fall, the arterioles dilate, and the blood flow through the organ appropriately increases.

Many substances in addition to oxygen are present within tissues and can affect the tone of the vascular smooth muscle. When the metabolic rate of skeletal muscle is increased by exercise, for example, not only do tissue levels of oxygen decrease, but those of carbon dioxide, H^+, and K^+ increase. Muscle tissue osmolarity also increases during exercise. All these chemical alterations cause arteriolar dilation. In

---

[2] An important exception to this rule occurs in the pulmonary circulation and is discussed later in this chapter.

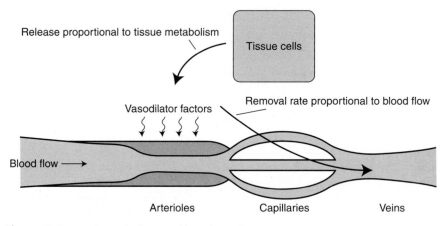

Figure 7–2. Local metabolic vasodilator hypothesis.

addition, with increased metabolic activity or oxygen deprivation, cells in many tissues may release *adenosine*, which is an extremely potent vasodilator agent.

At present, it is not known which of these (or possibly other) metabolically related chemical alterations within tissues are most important in the local metabolic control of blood flow. It appears likely that arteriolar tone depends on the combined action of many factors.

For conceptual purposes, Figure 7–2 summarizes current understanding of local metabolic control. Vasodilator factors enter the interstitial space from the tissue cells at a rate proportional to tissue metabolism. These vasodilator factors are removed from the tissue at a rate proportional to blood flow. Whenever tissue metabolism is proceeding at a rate for which the blood flow is inadequate, the interstitial vasodilator factor concentrations automatically build up and cause the arterioles to dilate. This, of course, causes blood flow to increase. The process continues until blood flow has risen sufficiently to appropriately match the tissue metabolic rate and prevent further accumulation of vasodilator factors. The same system also operates to reduce blood flow when it is higher than required by the tissue's metabolic activity, because this situation causes a reduction in the interstitial concentrations of metabolic vasodilator factors.

Local metabolic mechanisms represent by far the most important means of local flow control. By these mechanisms, individual organs are able to regulate their own flow in accordance with their metabolic needs. As indicated below, several other types of local influences on blood vessels have been identified. However, many of these represent fine-tuning mechanisms and many are important only in certain, usually pathological, situations.

LOCAL INFLUENCES FROM ENDOTHELIAL CELLS

Endothelial cells cover the entire inner surface of the cardiovascular system. A large number of studies have shown that blood vessels respond very differently to certain vascular influences when their endothelial lining is missing. Acetylcholine, for example, causes vasodilation of intact vessels but causes vasoconstriction of vessels stripped of their endothelial lining. This and similar results led to the realization that endothelial cells can actively participate in the control of arteriolar diameter by producing local chemicals that affect the tone of the surrounding smooth muscle cells. In the case of the vasodilator effect of infusing acetylcholine through intact vessels, the vasodilator influence produced by endothelial cells has been identified as nitric oxide. Nitric oxide is produced within endothelial cells from the amino acid, L-arginine, by the action of an enzyme, nitric oxide synthase. Nitric oxide synthase is activated by a rise in the intracellular level of the Ca^{2+}. Nitric oxide is a small lipid-soluble molecule that, once formed, easily diffuses into adjacent smooth muscle cells where it causes relaxation by stimulating cGMP production as mentioned previously.

Acetylcholine and several other agents (including bradykinin, vasoactive intestinal peptide, and substance P) stimulate endothelial cell nitric oxide production because their receptors on endothelial cells are linked to receptor-operated Ca^{2+} channels. Probably more importantly from a physiological standpoint, flow-related shear stresses on endothelial cells stimulate their nitric oxide production presumably because stretch-sensitive channels for Ca^{2+} are activated. Such flow-related endothelial cell nitric oxide production may explain why, for example, exercise and increased blood flow through muscles of the lower leg can cause dilation of the blood-supplying femoral artery at points far upstream of the exercising muscle itself.

Agents that block nitric oxide production by inhibiting nitric oxide synthase cause significant increases in the vascular resistances of most organs. For this reason, it is believed that endothelial cells are normally always producing some nitric oxide that is importantly involved, along with other factors, in reducing the normal net resting tone of arterioles throughout the body.

Endothelial cells have also been shown to produce several other locally acting vasoactive agents including the vasodilators "endothelial-derived hyperpolarizing factor" and prostacyclin and the vasoconstrictor *endothelin*. The roles of these agents in the overall scheme of normal checks and balances on local flow control are speculative at present. With the possible exception of flow-dependent, shear stress-related influences on endothelial cells, it is difficult to imagine how endothelial factors could play much of a role in tissue-specific blood flow control. The endothelial cells of arterioles in any organ are exposed primarily to the conditions in the incoming arterial blood rather than those in the tissues being served. Therefore, endothelial factors seem more likely to be important in global than local blood flow control.

OTHER LOCAL CHEMICAL INFLUENCES

In addition to local metabolic influences on vascular tone, many specific locally produced and locally acting chemical substances have been identified that have vascular effects and therefore could be important in local vascular regulation in certain instances. In most cases, however, definite information about the relative importance of these substances in cardiovascular regulation is lacking.

Prostaglandins and *thromboxane* are a group of several chemically related products of the cyclooxygenase pathway of arachidonic acid metabolism. Certain prostaglandins are potent vasodilators, while others are potent vasoconstrictors. Despite the vasoactive potency of the prostaglandins and the fact that most tissues (including endothelial cells and vascular smooth muscle cells) are capable of synthesizing prostaglandins, it has not been demonstrated convincingly that prostaglandins play a crucial role in *normal* vascular control. It is clear, however, that vasodilator prostaglandins are involved in inflammatory responses. Consequently, inhibitors of prostaglandin synthesis, such as aspirin, are effective anti-inflammatory drugs. Prostaglandins produced by platelets and endothelial cells are important in the hemostatic (flow stopping, antibleeding) vasoconstrictor and platelet-aggregating responses to vascular injury. Hence, aspirin is often prescribed to reduce the tendency for blood clotting—especially in patients with potential coronary flow limitations. Arachidonic acid metabolites produced via the lipoxygenase system (eg, *leukotrienes*) also have vasoactive properties and may influence blood flow and vascular permeability during inflammatory processes.

Histamine is synthesized and stored in high concentrations in secretory granules of tissue mast cells and circulating basophils. When released, histamine produces arteriolar vasodilation (via the cAMP pathway) and increases vascular permeability, which leads to edema formation and local tissue swelling. Histamine increases vascular permeability by causing separations in the junctions between the endothelial cells that line the vascular system. Histamine release is classically associated with *antigen–antibody reactions* in various allergic and immune responses. Many drugs and physical or chemical insults that damage tissue also cause histamine release. Histamine can stimulate sensory nerve endings to cause itching and pain sensations. While clearly important in many pathological situations, it seems unlikely that histamine participates in normal cardiovascular regulation.

Bradykinin is a small polypeptide that has about 10 times the vasodilator potency of histamine on a molar basis. It also acts to increase capillary permeability by opening the junctions between endothelial cells. Bradykinin is formed from certain plasma globulin substrates by the action of an enzyme, *kallikrein*, and is subsequently rapidly degraded into inactive fragments by various tissue kinases. Like histamine, bradykinin is thought to be involved in the vascular responses associated with tissue injury and immune reactions. It also stimulates nociceptive nerves and may thus be involved in the pain associated with tissue injury.

TRANSMURAL PRESSURE

The passive elastic mechanical properties of arteries and veins and how changes in transmural pressure affect their diameters were discussed in Chapter 6. The effect of transmural pressure on arteriolar diameter is more complex because arterioles respond both *passively* and *actively* to changes in transmural pressure. For example, a sudden increase in the internal pressure within an arteriole produces (1) first an initial slight passive mechanical distention (slight because arterioles are relatively thick-walled and muscular), and (2) then an active constriction that, within seconds, may completely reverse the initial distention. A sudden decrease in transmural pressure elicits essentially the opposite response, that is, an immediate passive decrease in diameter followed shortly by a decrease in active tone, which returns the arteriolar diameter to near that which existed before the pressure change. The active phase of such behavior is referred to as a *myogenic response*, because it seems to originate within the smooth muscle itself. The mechanism of the myogenic response is not known for certain, but stretch-sensitive ion channels on arteriolar vascular smooth muscle cells are likely candidates for involvement.

All arterioles have some normal distending pressure to which they are probably actively responding. Therefore, the myogenic mechanism is likely to be a fundamentally important factor in determining the basal tone of arterioles everywhere. Also, for obvious reasons and as soon discussed, the myogenic response is potentially involved in the vascular reaction to any cardiovascular disturbance that involves a change in arteriolar transmural pressure.

FLOW RESPONSES CAUSED BY LOCAL MECHANISMS

In organs with a highly variable metabolic rate, such as skeletal and cardiac muscles, the blood flow closely follows the tissue's metabolic rate. For example, skeletal muscle blood flow increases within seconds of the onset of muscle exercise and returns to control values shortly after exercise ceases. This phenomenon, which is illustrated in Figure 7–3A, is known as *exercise* or *active hyperemia* (*hyperemia* means high flow). It should be clear how active hyperemia could result from the local metabolic

Figure 7–3. Organ blood flow responses caused by local mechanisms: active and reactive hyperemias.

vasodilator feedback on the arteriolar smooth muscle. As alluded to previously, once initiated by local metabolic influences on small resistance vessels, endothelial flow-dependent mechanisms may assist in propagating the vasodilation to larger vessels upstream, which helps promote the delivery of blood to the exercising muscle.

Reactive or *postocclusion hyperemia* is a higher than normal blood flow that occurs transiently after the removal of any restriction that has caused a period of lower than normal blood flow. The phenomenon is illustrated in Figure 7–3B. For example, flow through an extremity is higher than normal for a period after a tourniquet is removed from the extremity. Both local metabolic and myogenic mechanisms may be involved in producing reactive hyperemia. The magnitude and duration of reactive hyperemia depend on the duration and severity of the occlusion as well as the metabolic rate of the tissue. These findings are best explained by an interstitial accumulation of metabolic vasodilator substances during the period of flow restriction. However, unexpectedly large flow increases can follow arterial occlusions lasting only 1 or 2 seconds. These may be explained best by a myogenic dilation response to the reduced intravascular pressure and decreased stretch of the arteriolar walls that exists during the period of occlusion.

Except when displaying active and reactive hyperemia, nearly all organs tend to keep their blood flow constant despite variations in arterial pressure—that is, they *autoregulate* blood flow. As shown in Figure 7–4A, an abrupt increase in arterial pressure is normally accompanied by an initial abrupt increase in organ blood flow that then gradually returns toward normal despite the sustained elevation in arterial pressure. The initial rise in flow with increased pressure is expected from the basic flow equation ($\dot{Q} = \Delta P/R$). The subsequent return of flow toward the normal level is caused by a gradual increase in active arteriolar tone and resistance to blood flow. Ultimately, a new steady state is reached with only slightly elevated blood flow because the increased driving pressure is counteracted by a higher than normal vascular resistance. As with the phenomenon of reactive hyperemia, blood flow autoregulation may be caused by both local metabolic feedback mechanisms and myogenic mechanisms. The arteriolar vasoconstriction responsible for the autoregulatory response shown in Figure 7–4A, for example, may be partially due to (1) a "washout" of metabolic vasodilator factors from the interstitium by the excessive initial blood flow and (2) a myogenic increase in arteriolar tone stimulated by the increase in stretching forces that the increase in pressure imposes on the vessel walls. There is also a *tissue pressure hypothesis* of blood flow autoregulation for which it is assumed that an abrupt increase in arterial pressure causes transcapillary fluid filtration and thus leads to a gradual increase in interstitial fluid volume and pressure. Presumably the increase in extravascular pressure would cause a decrease in vessel diameter by simple compression. This mechanism might be especially important in organs such as the kidney and brain whose volumes are constrained by external structures.

Although not illustrated in Figure 7–4A, autoregulatory mechanisms operate in the opposite direction in response to a decrease in arterial pressure below the normal value. One important general consequence of local autoregulatory mechanisms is that the steady-state blood flow in many organs tends to remain near the normal value over quite a wide range of arterial pressure. This is illustrated in the graph in Figure 7–4B. As discussed later, the inherent ability of certain organs to maintain

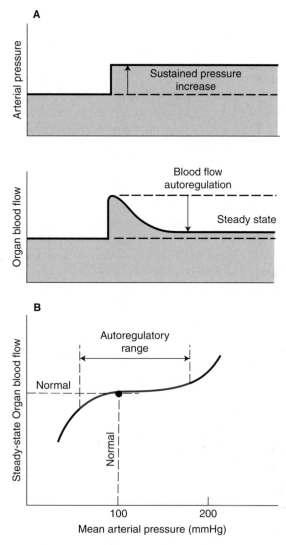

A

Arterial pressure

Sustained pressure
increase

Organ blood flow

Blood flow
autoregulation

Steady state

B

Steady-state Organ blood flow

Autoregulatory
range

Normal

Normal

100   200

Mean arterial pressure (mmHg)

Figure 7–4. Autoregulation of organ blood flow.

adequate blood flow despite lower than normal arterial pressure is of considerable importance in situations such as shock from blood loss.

Neural Influences on Arterioles

SYMPATHETIC VASOCONSTRICTOR NERVES

These neural fibers innervate arterioles in all systemic organs and provide by far the most important means of *reflex* control of the vasculature. Sympathetic vasoconstrictor nerves are the backbone of the system for controlling total peripheral resistance and thus are essential participants in global cardiovascular tasks such as regulating arterial blood pressure.

⑦ Sympathetic vasoconstrictor nerves release norepinephrine from their terminal structures in amounts generally proportional to their electrical activity. Norepinephrine causes an increase in the tone of arterioles after combining with an α_1-*adrenergic receptor* on smooth muscle cells. Norepinephrine appears to increase vascular tone primarily by pharmacomechanical means. The mechanism involves G-protein linkage of α-adrenergic receptors to phospholipase C and subsequent Ca^{2+} release from intracellular stores by the action of the second messenger IP_3, as illustrated in the right side of Figure 7–1.

Sympathetic vasoconstrictor nerves normally have a continual or *tonic firing activity*. This tonic activity of sympathetic vasoconstrictor nerves makes the normal contractile tone of arterioles considerably greater than their basal tone. The additional component of vascular tone is called *neurogenic tone*. When the firing rate of sympathetic vasoconstrictor nerves is increased above normal, arterioles constrict and cause organ blood flow to fall below normal. Conversely, vasodilation and increased organ blood flow can be caused by sympathetic vasoconstrictor nerves if their normal tonic activity level is reduced. Thus, an organ's blood flow can either be reduced below normal or be increased above normal by changes in the sympathetic vasoconstrictor fiber firing rate.

OTHER NEURAL INFLUENCES

Blood vessels, as a general rule, do not receive innervation from the parasympathetic division of the autonomic nervous system. However, *parasympathetic vasodilator nerves*, which release *acetylcholine*, are present in the vessels of the brain and the heart, but their influence on arteriolar tone in these organs appears to be inconsequential. Parasympathetic vasodilator nerves are also present in the vessels of the salivary glands, pancreas, gastric mucosa, and external genitalia. In the latter, they are responsible for the vasodilation of inflow vessels responsible for erection.

Hormonal Influences on Arterioles

⑤ Under normal circumstances, hormonal influences on blood vessels are generally thought to be of minor consequence in comparison to the local metabolic and neural influences. However, it should be emphasized that the understanding of how the cardiovascular system operates in many situations is incomplete. Thus, the hormones discussed in the following sections may play more important roles in cardiovascular regulation than is now appreciated.

CIRCULATING CATECHOLAMINES

During activation of the sympathetic nervous system, the adrenal glands release the catecholamines *epinephrine* and *norepinephrine* into the bloodstream. Under normal circumstances, the blood levels of these agents are probably not high enough to cause significant cardiovascular effects. However, circulating catecholamines may have cardiovascular effects in situations (such as vigorous exercise or hemorrhagic shock) that involve high activity of the sympathetic nervous system. In general, the cardiovascular effects of high levels of circulating catecholamines parallel the direct effects of sympathetic activation, which have already been discussed; both epinephrine and norepinephrine can activate cardiac β_1-adrenergic receptors to increase the heart rate and myocardial contractility and can activate vascular α-receptors to cause vasoconstriction. Recall that in addition to the α_1-receptors that mediate vasoconstriction, arterioles in a few organs also possess β_2-adrenergic receptors that mediate vasodilation. Because vascular β_2-receptors are more sensitive to epinephrine than are vascular α_1-receptors, moderately elevated levels of circulating epinephrine can cause vasodilation, whereas higher levels cause α_1-receptor-mediated vasoconstriction. Vascular β_2-receptors are not innervated and therefore are *not* activated by norepinephrine, released from sympathetic vasoconstrictor nerves. The physiological importance of these vascular β_2-receptors is unclear because adrenal epinephrine release occurs during periods of increased sympathetic activity when arterioles would simultaneously be undergoing direct neurogenic vasoconstriction. Again, under normal circumstances, circulating catecholamines are not an important factor in cardiovascular regulation.

VASOPRESSIN

This polypeptide hormone, also known as antidiuretic hormone, plays an important role in extracellular fluid homeostasis and is released into the bloodstream from the posterior pituitary gland in response to low blood volume and/or high extracellular fluid osmolarity. Vasopressin acts on collecting ducts in the kidneys to decrease renal excretion of water. Its role in body fluid balance has some very important indirect influences on cardiovascular function, which is discussed in more detail in Chapter 9. Vasopressin, however, is also a potent arteriolar vasoconstrictor. Although it is not thought to be significantly involved in normal vascular control, direct vascular constriction from abnormally high levels of vasopressin may be important in the response to certain disturbances such as severe blood loss through hemorrhage.

ANGIOTENSIN II

Angiotensin II is a circulating polypeptide that regulates aldosterone release from the adrenal cortex as part of the system for controlling body's sodium balance. This system, discussed in greater detail in Chapter 9, is very important in blood volume regulation. Angiotensin II is also a very potent vasoconstrictor agent. Although it should not be viewed as a normal regulator of arteriolar tone, direct vasoconstriction from angiotensin II seems to be an important component of the general cardiovascular response to severe blood loss. There is also strong evidence suggesting that direct vascular actions of angiotensin II may be involved in intrarenal mechanisms for controlling kidney function. In addition, angiotensin II may be partially responsible for the abnormal vasoconstriction that accompanies many forms of hypertension. Again, it should be emphasized that knowledge of many pathological situations—including hypertension—is incomplete. These situations may well involve vascular influences that are not yet recognized.

CONTROL OF VENOUS TONE

Before considering the details of the control of venous tone, recall that venules and veins play a much different role in the cardiovascular system than do arterioles. Arterioles are the inflow valves that control the rate of nutritive blood flow through organs and individual regions within them. Appropriately, arterioles are usually strongly influenced by the current local metabolic needs of the region in which they reside, whereas veins are not. Veins do, however, collectively regulate the distribution of available blood volume between the peripheral and central venous compartments. Recall that central blood volume (and therefore pressure) has a marked influence on stroke volume and cardiac output. Consequently, when one considers what *peripheral* veins are doing, one should be thinking primarily about what the effects will be on *central* venous pressure and cardiac output.

 Veins contain the vascular smooth muscle that is influenced by many things that influence the vascular smooth muscle of arterioles. Constriction of the veins (venoconstriction) is largely mediated through activity of the sympathetic nerves that innervate them. As in arterioles, these sympathetic nerves release norepinephrine, which interacts with α_1-receptors and produces an increase in venous tone and a decrease in vessel diameter. There are, however, several functionally important differences between veins and arterioles. Compared with arterioles, veins normally have little basal tone. Thus, veins are normally in a dilated state. One important consequence of the lack of basal venous tone is that vasodilator metabolites that may accumulate in the tissue have little effect on veins.

Because of their thin walls, veins are much more susceptible to physical influences than are arterioles. The large effect of internal venous pressure on venous diameter is discussed in Chapter 6 and is evident in the pooling of blood in the veins of the lower extremities that occurs during prolonged standing (as discussed further in Chapter 10).

Often external compressional forces are an important determinant of venous volume. This is especially true of veins in the skeletal muscle. Very high pressures are developed inside skeletal muscle tissue during contraction and cause venous vessels to collapse. Because veins and venules have one-way valves, the blood displaced from veins during skeletal muscle contraction is forced in the forward direction toward the right side of the heart. In fact, rhythmic skeletal muscle contractions can produce a considerable pumping action, often called the *skeletal muscle pump*, which helps return blood to the heart during exercise.

SUMMARY OF PRIMARY VASCULAR CONTROL MECHANISMS

As is apparent from the previous discussion, vessels are subject to a wide variety of influences, and special influences and/or situations often apply to particular organs. Certain general factors, however, dominate the primary control of the peripheral vasculature when it is viewed from the standpoint of overall cardiovascular system function; these influences are summarized in Figure 7–5. Basal tone, local

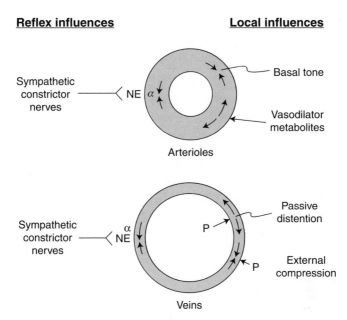

Reflex influences   **Local influences**

Arterioles

Veins

Figure 7–5. Primary influences on arterioles and veins. NE, norepinephrine; α, alpha-adrenergic receptor; P, pressure.

metabolic vasodilator factors, and sympathetic vasoconstrictor nerves acting through α_1-receptors are the major factors controlling arteriolar tone and therefore the blood flow rate through peripheral organs. Sympathetic vasoconstrictor nerves, internal pressure, and external compressional forces are the most important influences on venous diameter and therefore on peripheral–central distribution of blood volume. As evident in the remaining sections of this chapter, many details of vascular control vary from organs to organs. However, with regard to flow control, most organs can be placed somewhere in a spectrum that ranges from almost total dominance by local metabolic mechanisms to almost total dominance by sympathetic vasoconstrictor nerves.

The flow in organs such as the brain, heart muscle, and skeletal muscle is very strongly controlled by local metabolic control, whereas the flow in the kidneys, skin, and splanchnic organs is very strongly controlled by sympathetic nerve activity. Consequently, some organs are automatically forced to participate in overall cardiovascular reflex responses to a greater extent than are other organs. The overall plan seems to be that, in cardiovascular emergency, flow to the brain and heart will be preserved at the expense of everything else if need be.

VASCULAR CONTROL OF CORONARY BLOOD FLOW

The major right and left coronary arteries that serve the heart tissue are the first vessels to branch off the aorta. Thus, the driving force for myocardial blood flow is the systemic arterial pressure, just as it is for other systemic organs. Most of the blood that flows through the myocardial tissue returns to the right atrium by way of a large cardiac vein called the *coronary sinus.*

Local Metabolic Control

As emphasized before, coronary blood flow is controlled primarily by local metabolic mechanisms and thus it responds rapidly and accurately to changes in myocardial oxygen consumption. In a resting individual, the myocardium extracts 70 to 75% of the oxygen in the blood that passes through it. Coronary sinus blood normally has a lower oxygen content than blood at any other place in the cardiovascular system. Myocardial oxygen extraction cannot increase significantly from its resting value. Consequently, increases in myocardial oxygen consumption must be accompanied by appropriate increases in coronary blood flow.

The issue of *which* metabolic vasodilator factors play the dominant role in modulating the tone of coronary arterioles is unresolved at present. Many believe that adenosine, released from myocardial muscle cells in response to increased metabolic rate, may be an important local coronary metabolic vasodilator influence. Regardless of the specific details, myocardial oxygen consumption is the most important influence on coronary blood flow.

Systolic Compression

Large forces and/or pressures are generated *within* the myocardial tissue during cardiac muscle contraction. Such intramyocardial forces press on the outside of coronary vessels and cause them to collapse during systole. Because of this *systolic compression* and the associated collapse of coronary vessels, coronary vascular resistance is greatly increased during systole. The result, at least for much of the left ventricular myocardium, is that coronary flow is lower during systole than during diastole, even though systemic arterial pressure (ie, coronary perfusion pressure) is highest during systole. This is illustrated in the left coronary artery flow trace shown in Figure 7–6. Systolic compression has much less effect on flow through the right ventricular myocardium, as is evident from the right coronary artery flow trace in Figure 7–6. This is because the peak systolic intraventricular pressure is much lower for the right heart than for the left heart, and the systolic compressional forces in the right ventricular wall are correspondingly less than those in the left ventricular wall.

Systolic compressional forces on coronary vessels are greater in the endocardial (inside) layers of the left ventricular wall than in the epicardial layers.[3] Thus, the flow to the endocardial layers of the left ventricle is impeded more than the flow to epicardial layers by systolic compression. Normally, the endocardial region of the myocardium can make up for the lack of flow during systole by a high flow in the diastolic interval. However, when coronary blood flow is limited—for example, by

---

[3] Consider that the endocardial surface of the left ventricle is exposed to intraventricular pressure ($\simeq$120 mmHg during systole), while the epicardial surface is exposed only to intrathoracic pressure ($\simeq$0 mmHg).

Figure 7–6. Phasic flows in the left and right coronary arteries in relation to aortic and left ventricular pressures.

coronary disease and stenosis—the endocardial layers of the left ventricle are often the first regions of the heart to have difficulty maintaining a flow sufficient for their metabolic needs. *Myocardial infarcts* (areas of tissue killed by lack of blood flow) occur most frequently in the endocardial layers of the left ventricle.

Neural Influences on Coronary Flow

Coronary arterioles are densely innervated with sympathetic vasoconstrictor fibers, yet when the activity of the sympathetic nervous system increases, the coronary arterioles normally vasodilate rather than vasoconstrict. This is because an increase in sympathetic tone increases myocardial oxygen consumption by increasing the heart rate and contractility. The increased local metabolic vasodilator influence apparently outweighs the concurrent vasoconstrictor influence due to an increase in the activity of sympathetic vasoconstrictor fibers that terminate on coronary arterioles. It has been experimentally demonstrated that a given increase in cardiac sympathetic nerve activity causes a greater increase in coronary blood flow after the direct vasoconstrictor influence of sympathetic nerves on coronary vessels has been eliminated with α-receptor blocking agents. However, sympathetic vasoconstrictor nerves do not appear to influence coronary flow enough to affect the mechanical performance of normal hearts. Whether these coronary vasoconstrictor fibers might be functionally important in certain pathological situations is an open question.

VASCULAR CONTROL IN SPECIFIC ORGANS

The material presented in the rest of this chapter is perhaps most useful when considering the overall physiological characteristics of the specific organ or organ system. However, to give an overview of some of the vascular adaptations that can exist, the most important and/or unique circulatory characteristics for some major organs or organ systems are itemized in the following sections.

Skeletal Muscle Blood Flow

1. *Because of the large mass of the skeletal muscle, blood flow through it is an important factor in overall cardiovascular hemodynamics.* Collectively, the skeletal muscles constitute 40 to 45% of body weight—more than any other single body organ. Even at rest, approximately 15% of the cardiac output goes to skeletal muscle, and during strenuous exercise the skeletal muscle may receive more than 80% of the cardiac output.

2. *Resting skeletal muscle has a high level of intrinsic vascular tone.* Because of this high tone of the smooth muscle in resistance vessels of resting skeletal muscles, the blood flow per gram of tissue is quite low when compared with that of other organs such as the kidneys. However, resting skeletal muscle blood flow is still substantially above that required to sustain its metabolic needs. Resting skeletal muscles normally extract only 25 to 30% of the oxygen delivered to them in arterial blood. Thus, changes in the activity of sympathetic vasoconstrictor fibers can reduce resting muscle blood flow without compromising resting tissue metabolic processes.

3. *Local metabolic control of arteriolar tone is the most important influence on blood flow through exercising muscle.* A particularly important characteristic of skeletal muscle is its very wide range of metabolic rates. During heavy exercise, the oxygen consumption rate of and oxygen extraction by skeletal muscle tissue can reach the high values typical of the myocardium. In most respects, the factors that control blood flow to exercising muscle are similar to those that control coronary blood flow. Local metabolic control of arteriolar tone is very strong in exercising skeletal muscle, and muscle oxygen consumption is the most important determinant of its blood flow. Blood flow in the skeletal muscle can increase 20-fold during a bout of strenuous exercise.

4. *Alterations in sympathetic neural activity can alter non exercising skeletal muscle blood flow.* For example, maximum sympathetic discharge rates can decrease blood flow in a resting muscle to less than one-fourth its normal value, and conversely, if all neurogenic tone is removed, resting skeletal muscle blood flow may double. This is a modest increase in flow compared

what can occur in an exercising skeletal muscle. Nonetheless, because of the large mass of tissue involved, changes in the vascular resistance of resting skeletal muscle brought about by changes in sympathetic activity are very important in the overall reflex regulation of arterial pressure.

5. *Alterations in sympathetic neural activity can influence exercising skeletal muscle blood flow.* As discussed in Chapter 10, the cardiovascular response to muscle exercise involves a general increase in sympathetic activity. This of course reduces flow to susceptible organs, which include non exercising muscles. In exercising muscles, the increased sympathetic vasoconstrictor nerve activity is not evident as outright vasoconstriction but does limit the degree of metabolic vasodilation. One important function that this seemingly counterproductive process may serve is that of preventing an excessive reduction in total peripheral resistance during exercise. Indeed, if arterioles in most of the skeletal muscles in the body were allowed to dilate to their maximum capacity simultaneously, total peripheral resistance would be so low that the heart could not possibly supply enough cardiac output to maintain arterial pressure.

6. *Rhythmic contractions can increase venous return from exercising skeletal muscle.* As in the heart, muscle contraction produces large compressional forces within the tissue, which can collapse vessels and impede blood flow. Strong, sustained (tetanic) skeletal muscle contractions may actually stop muscle blood flow. Approximately 10% of the total blood volume is normally contained within the veins of the skeletal muscle, and during rhythmic exercise the "skeletal muscle pump" is very effective in displacing blood from skeletal muscle veins. Valves in the veins prevent reverse flow back into the muscles. Blood displaced from the skeletal muscle into the central venous pool is an important factor in the hemodynamics of strenuous whole body exercise.

7. *Veins in skeletal muscle can constrict in response to increased sympathetic activity.* However, veins in the skeletal muscle are rather sparsely innervated with sympathetic vasoconstrictor fibers, and the rather small volume of blood that can be mobilized from the skeletal muscle by sympathetic nerve activation is probably not of much significance to total body hemodynamics. This is in sharp contrast to the large displacement of blood from exercising muscle by the muscle pump mechanism. (This is discussed in more detail when postural reflexes are considered in Chapter 10.)

Cerebral Blood Flow

1. *Interruption of cerebral blood flow for more than a few seconds leads to unconsciousness and to brain damage within a very short period.* One rule of overall cardiovascular system function is that, in *all* situations, measures are taken that are appropriate to preserve adequate blood flow to the brain.

2. *Cerebral blood flow is regulated almost entirely by local mechanisms.* The brain as a whole has a nearly constant rate of metabolism that, on a per gram basis, is nearly as high as that of myocardial tissue. Flow through the cerebrum is

autoregulated very strongly and is little affected by changes in arterial pressure unless it falls below approximately 60 mmHg. When arterial pressure decreases below 60 mmHg, brain blood flow decreases proportionately. It is presently unresolved whether metabolic mechanisms or myogenic mechanisms or both are involved in the phenomenon of cerebral autoregulation.

3. *Local changes in cerebral blood flow may be influenced by local metabolic conditions.* Presumably because the overall average metabolic rate of brain tissue shows little variation, total brain blood flow is remarkably constant over nearly all situations. The cerebral activity in discrete locations within the brain, however, changes from situation to situation. As a result, blood flow to discrete regions is not constant but closely follows the local neuronal activity. The mechanisms responsible for this strong local control of cerebral blood flow are as yet undefined, but H^+, K^+, oxygen, and adenosine seem most likely to be involved.

4. *Cerebral blood flow decreases whenever arterial blood P_{CO_2} falls below normal.* Conversely, cerebral blood flow increases whenever the partial pressure of carbon dioxide (P_{CO_2}) is raised above normal in the arterial blood. This is the normal state of affairs in most tissues, but it plays out importantly when it happens in the brain. For example, the dizziness, confusion, and even fainting that can occur when a person hyperventilates (and "blows off" CO_2) are a direct result of cerebral vasoconstriction. It appears that cerebral arterioles respond not to changes in P_{CO_2} but to changes in the extracellular H^+ concentration (ie, pH) caused by changes in P_{CO_2}. Cerebral arterioles also vasodilate whenever the partial pressure of oxygen (P_{O_2}) in arterial blood falls significantly below normal values. However, higher than normal arterial blood P_{O_2}, such as that caused by pure oxygen inhalation, produces little decrease in cerebral blood flow.

5. *Sympathetic and parasympathetic neural influences on cerebral blood flow are minimal.* Although cerebral vessels receive both sympathetic vasoconstrictor and parasympathetic vasodilator fiber innervation, cerebral blood flow is influenced very little by changes in the activity of either under normal circumstances. Sympathetic vasoconstrictor responses may, however, be important in protecting cerebral vessels from excessive passive distention following large, abrupt increases in arterial pressure.

6. *The "blood–brain barrier" refers to the tightly connected vascular endothelial cells that severely restrict transcapillary movement of all polar and many other substances.*[4] Because of this blood–brain barrier, the extracellular space of the brain represents a special fluid compartment in which the chemical composition is regulated separately from that in the plasma and general body extracellular fluid compartment. The extracellular compartment of the brain encompasses both interstitial fluid and *cerebrospinal fluid* (CSF), which surrounds the brain and spinal cord and fills the brain ventricles. The CSF is formed from plasma by selective

---

[4] Brain capillaries have a special carrier system for glucose and present no barrier to oxygen and carbon dioxide diffusion. Thus, the blood–brain barrier does not restrict nutrient supply to the brain tissue.

secretion (not simple filtration) by specialized tissues, the *choroid plexes*, located within the ventricles. These processes regulate the chemical composition of the CSF. The interstitial fluid of the brain takes on the chemical composition of CSF through free diffusional exchange.

The blood–brain barrier serves to protect the cerebral cells from ionic disturbances in the plasma. Also, by exclusion and/or endothelial cell metabolism, it prevents many circulating hormones (and drugs) from influencing the parenchymal cells of the brain and the vascular smooth muscle cells in brain vessels.

Splanchnic Blood Flow

1. *Because of the high blood flow* through *and the high blood volume* in *the splanchnic bed, vascular control importantly influences overall cardiovascular hemodynamics.* A number of abdominal organs, including the gastrointestinal tract, spleen, pancreas, and liver, are collectively supplied with what is called the *splanchnic blood flow.* Splanchnic blood flow is supplied to these abdominal organs through many arteries, but it all ultimately passes through the liver and returns to the inferior vena cava through the hepatic veins. The organs of the splanchnic region receive approximately 25% of the resting cardiac output and moreover contain more than 20% of the circulating blood volume. Thus, adjustments in either the blood flow or the blood volume of this region have extremely important effects on the cardiovascular system.

2. *Sympathetic neural activity plays an important role in vascular control of the splanchnic circulation.* Collectively, the splanchnic organs have a relatively high blood flow and extract only 15 to 20% of the oxygen delivered to them in the arterial blood. The arteries and veins of all the organs involved in the splanchnic circulation are richly innervated with sympathetic vasoconstrictor nerves. Maximal activation of sympathetic vasoconstrictor nerves can produce an 80% reduction in flow to the splanchnic region and also cause a large shift of blood from the splanchnic organs to the central venous pool. In humans, a large fraction of the blood mobilized from the splanchnic circulation during periods of sympathetic activation comes from the constriction of veins in the liver. In many other species, the spleen acts as a major reservoir from which blood is mobilized by sympathetically mediated contraction of the smooth muscle located in the outer capsule of the organ.

3. *Local metabolic activity associated with motility, secretion, and absorption is associated with local increases in splanchnic blood flow.* There is a great diversity of function among individual organs and even regions within organs in the splanchnic region. The mechanisms of vascular control in specific areas of the splanchnic region are not well understood but are likely to be quite varied. Nonetheless, because most of the splanchnic organs are involved in the digestion and absorption of food from the gastrointestinal tract, splanchnic blood flow increases after food ingestion. A large meal can elicit a 30 to 100% increase

in splanchnic flow, but individual organs in the splanchnic region probably have higher percentage increases in flow at certain times because they are involved sequentially in the digestion–absorption process.

Renal Blood Flow

1. *Acute adjustments in renal blood flow have important hemodynamic consequences.* The kidneys normally receive approximately 20% of the cardiac output of a resting individual. This flow can be reduced to practically zero during strong sympathetic activation. Thus, the control of renal blood *flow* is important to overall cardiovascular function. However, because the kidneys are such small organs, changes in renal blood *volume* are inconsequential to overall cardiovascular hemodynamics.

2. *Renal blood flow is strongly influenced by sympathetic neural stimulation.* Alterations in sympathetic neural activity can have marked effects on total renal blood flow by altering the neurogenic tone of renal resistance vessels. In fact, extreme situations involving intense and prolonged sympathetic vasoconstrictor activity (as may accompany severe blood loss) can lead to dramatic reduction in renal blood flow, permanent kidney damage, and renal failure.

3. *Local mechanism may influence local vascular tone, but physiological roles are not clear.* It has long been known that experimentally *isolated* kidneys (ie, kidneys deprived of their normal sympathetic input) autoregulate their flow quite strongly. The mechanism responsible for this phenomenon has not been definitely established, but myogenic, tissue pressure, and metabolic hypotheses have been advanced. The real question is what purpose such a strong local mechanism plays in the intact organism where it seems to be largely overridden by reflex mechanisms. In an intact individual, renal blood flow is not constant but is highly variable, depending on the prevailing level of sympathetic vasoconstrictor nerve activity.

The mechanisms responsible for the intrinsic regulation of renal blood flow and kidney function have not been established. Although studies suggest that prostaglandins and some intrarenal renin–angiotensin system may be involved, the whole issue of local renal vascular control remains quite obscure. Renal function is itself of paramount importance to overall cardiovascular function, as described in Chapter 9.

Cutaneous Blood Flow

1. *The physiological role of skin blood flow is to help regulate body temperature.* The metabolic activity of body cells produces heat, which must be lost in order for the body temperature to remain constant. The skin is the primary site of exchange of body heat with the external environment. Alterations in cutaneous blood flow in response to various metabolic states and environmental conditions

provide the primary mechanism responsible for temperature homeostasis. (Other mechanisms such as shivering, sweating, and panting also participate in body temperature regulation under more extreme conditions.)

2. *Decreases in body temperature decrease skin blood flow and vice versa.* Cutaneous blood flow, which is about 6% of the resting cardiac output, can decrease to about one-twentieth of its normal value when heat is to be retained (eg, in a cold environment, during the development stages of a fever). In contrast, cutaneous blood flow can increase up to seven times its normal value when heat is to be lost (eg, in a hot environment, accompanying a high metabolic rate, after a fever "breaks").

3. *Structural adaptations of the cutaneous vascular beds promote heat loss or heat conservation.* The anatomic interconnections between microvessels in the skin are highly specialized and extremely complex. An extensive system of interconnected veins called the *venous plexus* normally contains the largest fraction of cutaneous blood volume, which, in individuals with lightly pigmented skin, gives the skin a reddish hue. To a large extent, heat transfer from the blood takes place across the large surface area of the venous plexus. The venous plexus is richly innervated with sympathetic vasoconstrictor nerves. When these fibers are activated, blood is displaced from the venous plexus, and this helps reduce heat loss and also lightens the skin color. Because the skin is one of the largest body organs, venous constriction can shift a considerable amount of blood into the central venous pool.

4. *Reflex sympathetic neural activity has important but complex influences on skin blood flow.* Cutaneous resistance vessels are richly innervated with sympathetic vasoconstrictor nerves, and because these fibers have a normal tonic activity, cutaneous resistance vessels normally have a high degree of neurogenic tone. When body temperature rises above normal, skin blood flow is increased by reflex mechanisms. In certain areas (such as the hands, ears, and nose), vasodilation appears to result entirely from the withdrawal of sympathetic vasoconstrictor tone. In other areas (such as the forearm, forehead, chin, neck, and chest), the cutaneous vasodilation that occurs with body heating greatly exceeds that which occurs with just the removal of sympathetic vasoconstrictor tone. This "active" vasodilation is closely linked to the onset of sweating in these areas. The sweat glands in human cutaneous tissue are innervated by *cholinergic sympathetic fibers* that release acetylcholine. Activation of these nerves elicits sweating *and* an associated marked cutaneous vasodilation. The exact mechanism for this sweating-related cutaneous vasodilation remains unclear because it is not abolished by agents that block acetylcholine's vascular effects. It has long been thought that it was caused by local bradykinin formation secondary to the process of sweat gland activation. Newer evidence suggests that the cholinergic sympathetic nerves to sweat glands may release not only acetylcholine but also other vasodilator cotransmitters. Although these special sympathetic nerves are very important to temperature regulation, they do not participate in the normal, moment-to-moment, regulation of the cardiovascular system.

5. *Cutaneous vessels respond to changes in local skin temperature.* In general, local cooling leads to local vasoconstriction and local heating causes local vasodilation. The mechanisms for this are unknown. If the hand is placed in ice water, there is initially a nearly complete cessation of hand blood flow accompanied by intense pain. After some minutes, hand blood flow begins to rise to reach values greatly in excess of the normal value, hand temperature increases, and the pain disappears. This phenomenon is referred to as *cold-induced vasodilation.* With continued immersion, hand blood flow cycles every few minutes between periods of essentially no flow and periods of hyperemia. The mechanism responsible for cold vasodilation is unknown, but it has been suggested that norepinephrine may lose its ability to constrict vessels when their temperature approaches 0°C. Whatever the mechanism, cold-induced vasodilation apparently serves to protect exposed tissues from cold damage.

6. *Cutaneous vessels respond to local damage with observable responses.* Tissue damage from burns, ultraviolet radiation, cold injury, caustic chemicals, and mechanical trauma produces reactions in skin blood flow. A classical reaction called the *triple response* is evoked after vigorously stroking the skin with a blunt point. The first component of the triple response is a *red line* that develops along the direct path of the abrasion in about 15 seconds. Shortly thereafter, an irregular *red flare* appears that extends about 2 cm on either side of the red line. Finally, after a minute or two, a *wheal* appears along the line of the injury. The mechanisms involved in the triple response are not well understood, but it seems likely that histamine release from damaged cells is at least partially responsible for the dilation evidenced by the red line and the subsequent edema formation of the wheal. The red flare seems to involve nerves in some sort of a local *axon reflex* because it can be evoked immediately after cutaneous nerves are sectioned but not after the peripheral portions of the sectioned nerves degenerate.

Pulmonary Blood Flow

1. *Pulmonary blood flow equals cardiac output.* The rate of blood flow through the lungs is necessarily equal to cardiac output in all circumstances. When cardiac output increases threefold during exercise, for example, pulmonary blood flow must also increase threefold. Although the flow through a systemic organ is determined by its vascular resistance ($\dot{Q} = \Delta P/R$), the blood flow rate through the lungs is determined simply by the cardiac output ($\dot{Q} = CO$).

2. *Pulmonary vascular resistance is about one-seventh of total systemic vascular resistance.* Pulmonary vessels do offer some vascular resistance. Although the level of pulmonary vascular resistance does not usually influence the pulmonary flow rate, it is important because it is one of the determinants of pulmonary arterial pressure ($\Delta P = \dot{Q} \times R$). Recall that mean *pulmonary* arterial pressure is approximately 13 mmHg, whereas mean *systemic* arterial pressure is approximately 100 mmHg. The reason for the difference in pulmonary and systemic arterial

pressures is not that the right side of the heart is weaker than the left side of the heart but rather that pulmonary vascular resistance is inherently much lower than systemic total peripheral resistance. The pulmonary bed has a low resistance because it has relatively large vessels throughout.

3. *Pulmonary arteries and arterioles are less muscular and more compliant than are systemic arteries and arterioles.* When pulmonary arterial pressure increases, the pulmonary arteries and arterioles become larger in diameter. Thus, an increase in pulmonary arterial pressure *decreases* pulmonary vascular resistance. This phenomenon is important because it tends to limit the increase in pulmonary arterial pressure that occurs with increases in cardiac output.

4. *Pulmonary arterioles constrict in response to local alveolar hypoxia.* One of the most important active responses in the pulmonary vasculature is the *hypoxic vasoconstriction* of pulmonary arterioles in response to low oxygen levels within the alveoli. This is exactly opposite to the vasodilation that occurs in systemic arterioles in response to low tissue P_{O_2}. The mechanisms that cause this unusual response in pulmonary vessels are unclear. Current evidence suggests that local prostaglandin synthesis may be involved in pulmonary hypoxic vasoconstriction. Whatever the mechanism, hypoxic vasoconstriction is essential to efficient lung gas exchange because it diverts blood flow away from areas of the lung that are underventilated. Consequently, the best-ventilated areas of the lung also receive the most blood flow. Presumably as a consequence of hypoxic arteriolar vasoconstriction, general hypoxia (such as that encountered at high altitude) causes an increase in pulmonary vascular resistance and pulmonary arterial hypertension.

5. *Autonomic nerves play no major role in control of pulmonary vascular activity.* Both pulmonary arteries and veins receive sympathetic vasoconstrictor fiber innervation, but reflex influences on pulmonary vessels appear to be much less important than the physical and local hypoxic influences. Pulmonary veins serve a blood reservoir function for the cardiovascular system, and sympathetic vasoconstriction of pulmonary veins may be important in mobilizing this blood during periods of general cardiovascular stress.

6. *Low capillary hydrostatic pressure promotes fluid reabsorption and prevents fluid accumulation in pulmonary airways.* A consequence of the low mean pulmonary arterial pressure is the low pulmonary capillary hydrostatic pressure of approximately 8 mmHg (compared with approximately 25 mmHg in systemic capillaries). Because the plasma oncotic pressure in lung capillaries is near 25 mmHg, as it is in all capillaries, it is likely that the transcapillary forces in the lungs strongly favor continual fluid reabsorption. This cannot be the complete story, however, because the lungs, like other tissues, continually produce some lymph and some net capillary filtration is required to produce lymphatic fluid. This filtration is possible despite the unusually low pulmonary capillary hydrostatic pressure because pulmonary interstitial fluid has an unusually high protein concentration and thus oncotic pressure.

KEY CONCEPTS

 Continual adjustments of vascular diameter are required to properly distribute the cardiac output to the various systemic tissues (the role of arterioles) and maintain adequate cardiac filling (the role of veins).

 Vascular adjustments are made by changes in the tone of the vascular smooth muscle.

 The vascular smooth muscle has many unique properties that make it sensitive to a wide array of local and reflex stimuli and capable of maintaining tone for long periods.

 The tone of arterioles, but not veins, can be strongly influenced by local vasodilator factors produced by local tissue metabolism.

 In abnormal situations (such as tissue injury or severe blood volume depletion), certain local factors such as histamine and bradykinin, and hormonal factors such as vasopressin and angiotensin have significant vascular influences.

 Sympathetic vasoconstrictor nerves provide the primary reflex mechanisms for regulating both arteriolar and venous tones.

 Sympathetic vasoconstrictor nerves release norepinephrine, which interacts with α_1-adrenergic receptors on the vascular smooth muscle to induce vasoconstriction.

 The relative importance of local metabolic versus reflex sympathetic control of arteriolar tone (and therefore blood flow) varies from organs to organs.

 In some organs (such as the brain, heart muscle, and exercising skeletal muscle), blood flow normally closely follows metabolic rate because of local metabolic influences on arterioles.

 In other organs (such as skin and kidneys), blood flow is normally regulated more by sympathetic nerves than by local metabolic conditions.

 STUDY QUESTIONS

7–1. Which of the following would increase blood flow through a skeletal muscle?
   a. an increase in tissue P_{CO_2}
   b. an increase in tissue adenosine
   c. the presence of α-receptor-blocking drugs
   d. sympathetic activation

7-2. Autoregulation of blood flow implies that arterial pressure is adjusted by local mechanisms to ensure constant flow through an organ. True or false?

7-3. Coronary blood flow will normally increase when
    a. arterial pressure increases
    b. the heart rate increases
    c. sympathetic activity increases
    d. the heart is dilated

7-4. The arterioles of skeletal muscle would have little or no tone in the absence of normal sympathetic vasoconstrictor fiber activity. True or false?

7-5. A person who hyperventilates (breathes rapidly and deeply) gets dizzy. Why?

7-6. A patient complains of severe leg pains after walking a short distance. The pains disappear after the patient rests. (This symptom is called intermittent claudication.) What might be the problem?

7-7. How would a stenotic aortic valve influence coronary blood flow?

7-8. Vascular smooth muscle differs from cardiac muscle in that it
    a. contains no actin molecules
    b. can be directly activated in the absence of action potentials
    c. is unresponsive to changes in intracellular calcium levels
    d. is unresponsive to changes in membrane potentials
    e. is unresponsive to changes in muscle length

7-9. Arteriolar constriction tends to do which of the following?
    a. decrease total peripheral resistance
    b. decrease mean arterial pressure
    c. decrease capillary hydrostatic pressure
    d. increase transcapillary fluid filtration
    e. increase blood flow through the capillary bed

7-10. When an organ responds to an increase in metabolic activity with a decrease in arteriolar resistance, this is known as
    a. active hyperemia
    b. reactive hyperemia
    c. autoregulation of blood flow
    d. flow-dependent vasodilation
    e. metabolic vasoconstriction

Central Venous Pressure: An Indicator of Circulatory Hemodynamics

8

OBJECTIVES

The student understands how central venous pressure can be used to assess circulatory states and how venous return, cardiac output, and central venous pressure are interrelated:

▶ *Describes the overall arrangement of the systemic circulation and identifies the primary functional properties of each of its major components.*

▶ *Defines mean circulatory filling pressure and states the primary factors that determine it.*

▶ *Defines venous return and explains how it is distinguished from cardiac output.*

▶ *States the reason why cardiac output and venous return must be equal in the steady state.*

▶ *Lists the factors that control venous return.*

▶ *Describes the relationship between central venous pressure and venous return and draws the normal venous return curve.*

▶ *Defines peripheral venous pressure.*

▶ *Lists the factors that determine peripheral venous pressure.*

▶ *Predicts the shifts in the venous return curve that occur with altered blood volume and altered venous tone.*

▶ *Describes how the output of the left heart pump is matched to that of the right heart pump.*

▶ *Draws the normal venous return and cardiac output curves on a graph and describes the significance of the point of curve intersection.*

▶ *Predicts how normal venous return, cardiac output, and central venous pressure will be altered with any given combination of changes in cardiac sympathetic tone, peripheral venous sympathetic tone, or circulating blood volume.*

▶ *Identifies possible conditions that result in abnormally high or low central venous pressure.*

INTERACTION OF SYSTEM COMPONENTS

Once one has learned the basic facts concerning the individual pieces of the cardiovascular system, it is important to step back, take a broad view, and see how those pieces interact in the operation of the intact system.

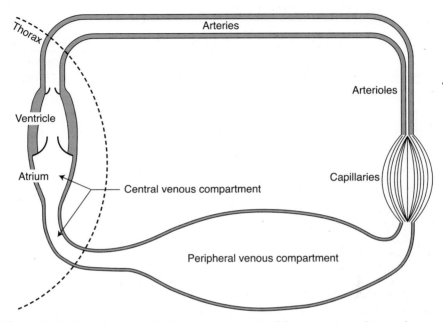

Figure 8–1. Major functionally distinct components of the systemic cardiovascular circuit.

As illustrated in Figure 8–1, the cardiovascular system is a closed hydraulic circuit that includes the heart, arteries, arterioles, capillaries, and veins.[1] The venous side of this system is often conceptually separated into two different compartments: (1) a large and diverse peripheral section (the peripheral venous compartment) and (2) a smaller intrathoracic section that includes the vena cavae and the right atrium (the central venous compartment). Each of the segments of this circuit has a distinctly different role to play in the overall operation of the system because of inherent differences in anatomical volume, resistance to flow, and compliance that are summarized in Table 8–1.

Note especially the surprisingly high ventricular diastolic compliance of 24 mL/mmHg in Table 8–1. This value indicates how exquisitely sensitive the ventricular end-diastolic volume (and therefore stroke volume and cardiac output) is to small changes in cardiac filling pressure (ie, central venous pressure). In all physiological and pathological situations, cardiac filling pressure is a crucial factor that determines how well the cardiovascular system will be operating.

---

[1] The pulmonary circuit is not included in Figure 8–1 because it does not influence the major points to be made in this chapter. The primary leap of faith in this omission is that, because of Starling's law of the heart, changes in the end-diastolic volume of the *right* ventricle cause equal changes in the end-diastolic volume of the *left* ventricle.

Table 8–1. Typical Properties of the Major Components of the Systemic Cardiovascular Circuit*

Compartment	V_0 (mL)	C (mL/mmHg)	R (mmHg/L per minute)
Ventricle in diastole	30	24	0
Arteries	600	2	1
Arterioles	100	0	13
Capillaries	250	0	5
Peripheral venous compartment	2500	110	1
Central venous compartment	80	4	0
Entire circuit	3560	140	20

*Values are for a normal, young, resting 70-kg adult.
V_0, anatomical volume of compartment at zero pressure; C, compliance of compartment; R, resistance to flow through compartment.

Mean Circulatory Filling Pressure

Imagine the heart arrested in diastole with no flow around the circuit shown in Figure 8–1. It will take a certain amount of blood just to fill the anatomical space contained by the systemic system without stretching any of its walls or developing any internal pressure. This amount is 3.56 L, as indicated by the total systemic circuit volume (V_0) in Table 8–1. Normally, however, the systemic circuit contains approximately 4.5 L of blood and thus is somewhat inflated. From the total systemic circuit compliance (C) given in Table 8–1, one can see that an extra 1000 mL of blood would result in an internal pressure of approximately 7 mmHg (ie, 1000 mL/140 mL per mmHg). This theoretical pressure is called the *mean circulatory filling pressure* and is the actual pressure that would exist throughout the system in the absence of flow.

 The two major variables that affect mean circulatory filling pressure are the circulating blood volume and the state of the peripheral venous vessel tone. In the latter case, look at Figure 8–1 and imagine how constriction of the vessels of the large venous compartment (increasing venous tone) will significantly increase pressure throughout the system. In contrast, squeezing on arterioles (increasing arteriolar tone) will have a negligible effect on mean circulatory filling pressure because arterioles contain so little blood in any state. The other major components of the system (arteries and capillaries) essentially do not actively change their volume.

Flow-Induced Distribution of Blood Volume and Pressure

The presence of flow around the circuit does not change the total volume of blood in the system or the mean circulatory filling pressure. The flow caused by cardiac pumping action does, however, tend to shift some of the blood volume from the venous side of the circuit to the arterial side. This causes pressures on the arterial side to rise above the mean circulatory pressure while pressures on the venous side fall below it. Because veins are about 50 times more compliant than arteries (Table 8–1), the flow-induced decrease in venous pressure is only about 1/50th as large as the accompanying increase in arterial pressure. Thus, flow or no flow, pressure in the peripheral venous compartment is normally quite close to the mean circulatory filling pressure.

CENTRAL VENOUS PRESSURE: AN INDICATOR OF CIRCULATORY STATUS

The cardiovascular system must adjust its operation continually to meet changing metabolic demands of the body. Because the cardiovascular system is a closed hydraulic loop, adjustments in any one part of the circuit will have pressure, flow, and volume effects throughout the circuit. Because of the critical influence of cardiac filling on cardiovascular function, the remainder of this chapter focuses on the factors that determine the pressure in the central venous compartment. In addition, the way in which measures of central venous pressure can provide clinically useful information about the state of the circulatory system is discussed.

The central venous compartment corresponds roughly to the volume enclosed by the right atrium and the great veins in the thorax. Blood *leaves* the central venous compartment by entering the right ventricle at a rate that is equal to the cardiac output. *Venous return*, in contrast, is by definition the rate at which blood returns to the thorax from the peripheral vascular beds and thus is the rate at which blood *enters* the central venous compartment. The important distinction between venous return *to* the central venous compartment and cardiac output *from* the central venous compartment is illustrated in Figure 8–2.

In any stable situation, venous return must equal cardiac output or blood would gradually accumulate in either the central venous compartment or the peripheral vasculature. However, there are often temporary differences between cardiac output and venous return. Whenever such differences exist, the volume of the central venous compartment must be changing. Because the central venous compartment is

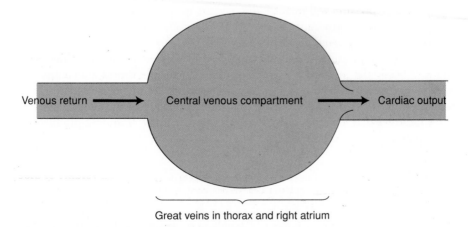

Venous return ➡ Central venous compartment ➡ Cardiac output

Great veins in thorax and right atrium

Figure 8–2. Distinction between cardiac output and venous return.

enclosed by elastic tissues, any change in central venous volume produces a corresponding change in central venous pressure.

As discussed in Chapter 3, the central venous pressure (ie, cardiac filling pressure) has an extremely important *positive* influence on stroke volume, and therefore, cardiac output (Starling's law of the heart). As argued later, central venous pressure has an equally important *negative* effect on venous return. Thus, central venous pressure is always automatically driven to a value that makes cardiac output equal to venous return. The factors that determine central venous pressure in any given situation are discussed in the following section.

INFLUENCE OF CENTRAL VENOUS PRESSURE ON VENOUS RETURN

The important factors involved in the process of venous return can be summarized as shown in Figure 8–3A. Basically, venous return is blood flow from the peripheral venous compartment to the central venous compartment through converging vessels. Anatomically the peripheral venous compartment is scattered throughout the systemic organs, but functionally it can be viewed as a single vascular space that has a particular pressure (P_{PV}) at any instant of time. The normal operating pressure in the peripheral venous compartment is usually very close to mean circulatory filling pressure. Moreover, the same factors that influence mean circulatory filling pressure have essentially equal influences on peripheral venous pressure. Thus "peripheral venous pressure" can be viewed as essentially equivalent to "mean circulatory filling pressure." The blood flow rate between the peripheral venous compartment and the central venous compartment is governed by the basic flow equation ($\dot{Q} = \Delta P/R$), where ΔP is the pressure drop between the peripheral and central venous compartments and R is the small resistance associated with the peripheral veins. In the example in Figure 8–3, peripheral venous pressure is assumed to be 7 mmHg. Thus, there will be no venous return when the central venous pressure (P_{CV}) is also 7 mmHg as shown in Figure 8–3B.

If the peripheral venous pressure remains at 7 mmHg, decreasing central venous pressure will increase the pressure drop across the venous resistance and consequently cause an elevation in venous return. This relationship is summarized by the *venous function curve*, which shows how venous return increases as central venous pressure drops.[2] If central venous pressure reaches very low values and falls below the intrathoracic pressure, the veins in the thorax are compressed which therefore tends to limit venous return. In the example in Figure 8–3, intrathoracic pressure is taken to be 0 mmHg and the flat portion of the venous function curve indicates that lowering central venous pressure below 0 mmHg produces no additional increase in venous return.

---

[2] The slope of the venous function curve is determined by the value of the venous vascular resistance. Lowering the venous vascular resistance would tend to raise the venous function curve and make it steeper because more venous return would result for a given difference between P_{PV} and P_{CV}. However, if P_{PV} is 7 mmHg, venous return will be 0 L/min when $P_{CV} = 7$ mmHg at any level of venous vascular resistance ($\dot{Q} = \Delta P/R$). We have chosen to ignore the complicating issue of changes in venous vascular resistance because they do not affect the general conclusions to be drawn from the discussion of venous function curves.

Figure 8–3. (**A**) Factors influencing venous return and (**B**) the venous function curve.

Just as a cardiac function curve shows how central venous pressure influences cardiac output, *a venous function curve shows how central venous pressure influences venous return.*[3]

INFLUENCE OF PERIPHERAL VENOUS PRESSURE ON VENOUS RETURN

As can be deduced from Figure 8–3A, it is the pressure difference between the peripheral and central venous compartments that determines venous return.

---

[3] Graphic relationships are almost invariably plotted with the *independent* variable on the horizontal axis (abscissa) and the *dependent* variable on the vertical axis (ordinate) and they *must* be read in that sense. For example, Figure 8–3B says that increasing central venous pressure tends to cause decreased venous return. Figure 8–3B *does not* imply that increasing venous return will tend to lower central venous pressure.

Therefore, an increase in peripheral venous pressure can be just as effective in increasing venous return as a drop in central venous pressure.

 The two ways in which peripheral venous pressure can change were discussed in Chapter 6. First, because veins are elastic vessels, changes in the *volume* of blood contained within the peripheral veins alter the peripheral venous pressure. Moreover, because the veins are much more compliant than any other vascular segment, changes in circulating blood volume produce larger changes in the volume of blood in the veins than in any other vascular segment. For example, blood loss by hemorrhage or loss of body fluids through severe sweating, vomiting, or diarrhea will decrease circulating blood volume and significantly reduce the volume of blood contained in the veins and thus decrease the peripheral venous pressure. Conversely, transfusion, fluid retention by the kidney, or transcapillary fluid reabsorption will increase circulating blood volume and venous blood volume. Whenever circulating blood volume increases, so does peripheral venous pressure.

 Recall from Chapter 7 that the second way that peripheral venous pressure can be altered is through changes in venous tone produced by increasing or decreasing the activity of sympathetic vasoconstrictor nerves supplying the venous smooth muscle. Peripheral venous pressure increases whenever the activity of sympathetic vasoconstrictor fibers to veins increases. In addition, an increase in any force compressing veins from the outside has the same effect on the pressure inside veins as an increase in venous tone. Thus, such things as muscle exercise and wearing elastic stockings tend to elevate peripheral venous pressure.

Whenever peripheral venous pressure is altered, the relationship between central venous pressure and venous return is also altered. For example, whenever peripheral venous pressure is elevated by increases in blood volume or by sympathetic stimulation, the venous function curve shifts upward and to the right (Figure 8–4). This phenomenon can be most easily understood by focusing first on the central venous pressure at which there will be no venous return. If peripheral venous pressure is 7 mmHg, then venous return will be 0 L/min when central venous pressure is 7 mmHg. If peripheral venous pressure is increased to 10 mmHg, then considerable venous return will occurs when central venous pressure is 7 mmHg, and venous return will stop only when central venous pressure is raised to 10 mmHg. Thus, increasing peripheral venous pressure shifts the whole venous function curve upward and to the right. By similar logic, decreased peripheral venous pressure caused by blood loss or decreased sympathetic vasoconstriction of peripheral veins shifts the venous function curve downward and to the left (Figure 8–4).

DETERMINATION OF CARDIAC OUTPUT AND VENOUS RETURN BY CENTRAL VENOUS PRESSURE

The significance of the fact that central venous pressure simultaneously affects both cardiac output and venous return can be best seen by plotting the cardiac function curve (the Starling curve) and the venous function curve on the same graph, as shown in Figure 8–5.

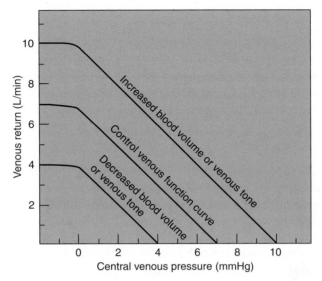

Figure 8–4. Effect of changes in blood volume and venous tone on venous function curves.

CVP ⤷ CO
⤷ VR)

PVP = Peripheral
Venous
Pressure

Figure 8–5. Interaction of cardiac output and venous return through central venous pressure.

Central venous pressure, as defined earlier, is the filling pressure of the right heart. Strictly speaking, this pressure directly affects only the stroke volume and output of the *right* heart pump. In most contexts, however, "cardiac output" implies the output of the *left* heart pump. How is it then, as has often been previously implied, that central venous pressure (the filling pressure of the right side of the heart) profoundly affects cardiac output (the output of the left side of the heart)? The short answer is that in the steady state, the right and left sides of the heart have equal outputs. (Because the right and left sides of the heart always beat with identical rates, this implies that their stroke volumes must be equal in the steady state.) The proper answer is that changes in central venous pressure automatically cause essentially parallel changes in the filling pressure of the left side of the heart (ie, in left atrial pressure). Consider, for example, the following sequence of consequences that a small step wise increase in central venous pressure has on a heart that previously was in a steady state:

1. Increased central venous pressure.
2. Increased right ventricular stroke volume via Starling's law.
3. Increased output of the right side of the heart.
4. The right side of the heart output temporarily exceeds that of the left side of the heart.
5. As long as this imbalance exists, blood accumulates in the pulmonary vasculature and raises pulmonary venous and left atrial pressures.
6. Increased left atrial pressure increases left ventricular stroke volume via Starling's law.
7. Very quickly, a new steady state will be reached when left atrial pressure has risen sufficiently to make left ventricular stroke volume exactly equal to the increased right ventricular stroke volume.

The major conclusion here is that left atrial pressure will automatically change in the correct direction to match left ventricular stroke volume to the current right ventricular stroke volume. Consequently, it is usually an acceptable simplification to say that central venous pressure affects cardiac output as if the heart consisted only of a single pump.

Note that in Figure 8–5, cardiac output and venous return are equal (at 5 L/min) *only* when the central venous pressure is 2 mmHg. If central venous pressure were to decrease to 0 mmHg for any reason, cardiac output would fall (to 2 L/min) and venous return would increase (to 7 L/min). With a venous return of 7 L/min and a cardiac output of 2 L/min, the volume of the central venous compartment would necessarily be increasing and this would produce a progressively increasing central venous pressure. In this manner, central venous pressure would return to the original level (2 mmHg) in a very short time. Moreover, if central venous pressure were to increase from 2 to 4 mmHg for any reason, venous return would decrease (to 3 L/min) and cardiac output would increase (to 7 L/min). This would quickly reduce the volume of blood in the central venous pool, and the central venous pressure would soon fall back to the original level. The cardiovascular system

Figure 8–6. Families of cardiac function and venous function curves. Intersection points indicate equilibrium values for cardiac output, venous return, and central venous pressure under various conditions.

automatically adjusts to operate at the point where the cardiac and venous function curves intersect.

Central venous pressure is always inherently driven to the value that makes cardiac output and venous return equal. Cardiac output and venous return always stabilize at the level where the cardiac function and venous function curves intersect.

In order to fulfill its homeostatic role in the body, the cardiovascular system must be able to alter its cardiac output. Recall from Chapter 3 that cardiac output is affected by more than just cardiac filling pressure and that at any moment the heart may be operating on any one of a number of cardiac function curves, depending on the existing level of cardiac sympathetic tone. The family of possible cardiac function curves may be plotted along with the family of possible venous function curves, as shown in Figure 8–6. At a particular moment, the existing influences on the heart dictate the particular cardiac function curve on which it is operating, and similarly, the existing influences on peripheral venous pressure dictate the particular venous function curve that applies. Thus, the influences on the heart and on the peripheral vasculature determine where the cardiac and venous function curves intersect and thus what the central venous pressure and cardiac output (and venous return) are in the steady state. In the intact cardiovascular system, cardiac output can rise only when the point of intersection of the cardiac and venous function curves is raised. *All changes in cardiac output are caused by a shift in the cardiac function curve, a shift in the venous function curve, or both.*

The cardiac function and venous function curves are useful for understanding the complex interactions that occur in the intact cardiovascular system. With the

$CO = SU \times HR$

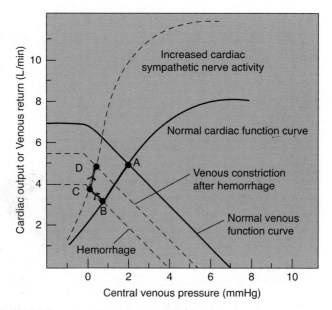

Figure 8–7. Cardiovascular adjustments to hemorrhage.

help of Figure 8–7, let us consider, for example, what happens to the cardiovascular system when there is a significant loss of blood (hemorrhage). Assume that before the hemorrhage, sympathetic activity to the heart and peripheral vessels is normal, as is the blood volume. Therefore, cardiac output is related to central venous pressure as indicated by the "normal" cardiac function curve in Figure 8–7. In addition, venous return is determined by central venous pressure as indicated by the "normal" venous function curve shown. The normal cardiac and venous function curves intersect at point A, so cardiac output is 5 L/min and central venous pressure is 2 mmHg in the normal state. When blood volume decreases because of hemorrhage, the peripheral venous pressure falls and the venous function curve is shifted to the left. In the absence of any cardiovascular responses, the cardiovascular system must switch its operation to point B because this is now the point at which the cardiac function curve and the new venous function curve intersect. This automatically occurs because, at the moment of blood loss, the venous function curve is shifted to the left and venous return falls below cardiac output at the central venous pressure of 2 mmHg. This is what leads to the fall in the central venous compartment's volume and pressure that causes the shift in operation from point A to point B. Note by comparing points A and B in Figure 8–7 that blood loss itself lowers cardiac output and central venous pressure by shifting the venous function curve. In going from point A to point B, cardiac output falls solely because of decreased filling pressure and Starling's law of the heart.

Subnormal cardiac output evokes a number of cardiovascular compensatory mechanisms to bring cardiac output back to more normal levels. One of these compensatory mechanisms is an increase in the activity of cardiac sympathetic nerves,

only to the Heart not vasculature

which, as discussed in Chapter 3, shifts the heart's operation to a cardiac function curve that is higher than normal. The effect of increasing cardiac sympathetic activity is illustrated by a shift in cardiovascular operation from point B to point C. In itself, the increased cardiac sympathetic nerve activity increases cardiac output (from 3 to 4 L/min) but causes a further decrease in central venous pressure. This drop in central venous pressure occurs because points B and C lie on the same venous function curve. *Cardiac* sympathetic nerves do not affect the venous function curve.[4]   ↑ Contractility ↑ SU ↑ CO

An additional compensatory mechanism evoked by blood loss is increased activity of the sympathetic nerves leading to veins. Recall that this raises peripheral venous pressure and causes a rightward shift of the venous function curve. Therefore, increased sympathetic activity to veins tends to shift the venous function curve, originally lowered by blood loss, back toward normal. As a consequence of the increased peripheral venous tone and the shift to a more normal venous function curve, the cardiovascular operation shifts from point C to point D in Figure 8–7. Thus, peripheral venous constriction increases cardiac output by raising central venous pressure and moving the heart's operation upward along a fixed cardiac function curve. It must be pointed out that separating the response to hemorrhage into distinct, progressive steps (ie, A to B to C to D) is only a conceptualization for appreciating the individual effects of the different processes involved. In reality, the reflex venous and cardiac responses occur simultaneously and so quickly that they will easily keep up with the blood loss as it occurs. Thus, the actual course of a patient's net response to hemorrhage would follow nearly a straight line from point A to point D.

In summary, point D illustrates that normal cardiac output can be sustained in the face of blood loss by the combined effect of peripheral and cardiac adjustments. Hemorrhage is only one of an almost infinite variety of disturbances to the cardiovascular system. Plots such as those shown in Figure 8–7 are very useful for understanding the many disturbances to the cardiovascular system and the ways in which they may be compensated.

CLINICAL IMPLICATIONS OF ABNORMAL CENTRAL VENOUS PRESSURES

Although, in the clinical situation, there is no way to actually determine the position of either cardiac function or venous function curves, important information about the patient's circulatory status can be obtained from measures of central venous pressure. From what has been presented in this chapter, it is possible to conclude that a patient with *abnormally high* central venous pressure must have a depressed cardiac function curve, a right-shifted venous function curve, or both. As discussed in Chapter 11, very high central venous pressures are a hallmark of patients with congestive heart failure because they have the combination of dysfunctional heart muscle (depressed cardiac function curve) *and* excessive

---

[4] Venous return is higher at point C than at point B, but the venous function *curve* has not shifted.

fluid volume (right-shifted venous function curve). *Abnormally low* central venous pressures, on the other hand, could theoretically be caused by either an elevated cardiac function curve or a left-shifted venous function curve. The clinical reality is that abnormally low central venous pressures are invariably the result of a left shift of the venous function curve, caused by either low blood volume or lack of venous tone.

Rough estimates of a patient's central venous pressure can be obtained quite easily by observing the external jugular veins. Because the force of gravity tends to keep veins in the head and neck collapsed when an individual is in an upright position, there should be no distention (or retrograde pulsations from atrial contractions) observed in these neck veins. Conversely, when an individual is fully recumbent, the neck veins should be full and pulsations should be easily detected. If a healthy individual is placed in a semirecumbent position so that the external jugular veins are positioned at ~7 cm above the right atrium, the point between the collapsed venous segment and the filled segment can usually be visualized.[5] Abnormally high central venous pressures will be associated with neck vein distention at a higher level (perhaps even when the patient is upright).

Because of its diagnostic value in critical care situations, central venous pressure is often monitored continuously via a catheter that is inserted in a peripheral vein and advanced centrally until its tip is in the central venous compartment (ie, near or in the right atrium). In some situations, it is desirable to assess *left atrial* pressure, which is the filling pressure for the left side of the heart. This is commonly done with a specialized flow-directed venous catheter that uses a small inflatable balloon at its tip to drag it with the blood flow through the right ventricle and pulmonic valve into the pulmonary artery. The balloon is then deflated and the cannula is advanced further until it wedges into a terminal branch of the pulmonary vasculature. The *pulmonary wedge pressure* recorded at this junction provides a useful estimate of left atrial pressure.

I V Cardiology Baby!!

KEY CONCEPTS

Mean circulatory filling pressure is a theoretical measure of pressure in the systemic circuit when flow is stopped and is influenced primarily by blood volume and peripheral venous tone.

Central venous pressure has a negative influence on venous return that can be illustrated graphically as a venous function curve.

---

[5] The astute reader will note that 7-cm H_2O is equal to about 5 mmHg. This is significantly higher than the 2-mmHg central venous pressure we have used for argument elsewhere in this text. As discussed in Chapter 10, gravity causes body position-dependent shifts of blood volume between the peripheral and central venous pools. Thus, central venous pressure is normally higher in the recumbent than in the upright position.

Peripheral venous pressure has a positive influence on venous return and can be elevated by increased blood volume and/or increased venous tone.

 Because of its opposing influences on cardiac output and venous return, central venous pressure automatically assumes a value that makes cardiac output and venous return equal.

Central venous pressure gives clinically relevant information about circulatory status.

 Central venous pressure can be estimated noninvasively by noting the fullness of a patient's jugular veins.

STUDY QUESTIONS

[handwritten: Decrease in arteriolar tone isn't Sufficient enough to influence MCFP or MCV]
[handwritten: Influence Factors – Blood volume – PVP]

8–1. Which of the following will *decrease* the mean circulatory filling pressure?
    a. increased circulating blood volume
    b. decreased arteriolar tone *[handwritten: none are correct]*
    c. increased venous tone

8–2. What determines *central venous pressure*? *[handwritten: Venous Return, Peripheral Venous Pressure, Volume, tone, Cardiac Output]*

8–3. According to Starling's law, cardiac output always decreases when central venous pressure decreases. True or false? *[handwritten: CO↓ ← CVP↓]*

8–4. In a steady state, venous return will be greater than cardiac output when *[handwritten: Steady State VR=CO]*
    a. peripheral venous pressure is higher than normal
    b. blood volume is higher than normal
    c. cardiac sympathetic nerve activity is lower than normal *[handwritten: ↓CO ↓CVP = Preload]*

8–5. What approaches might a physician logically pursue in an attempt to lower a patient's cardiac preload? *[handwritten: Diurese to pull Blood volume off, Digoxin ↑ CO]*

8–6. In a severely dehydrated patient, you would expect to find *[handwritten: ↓ Blood volume]*
    a. a depressed cardiac function curve *[handwritten: ↓PVP → ↓VR > ↓CVP]*
    b. an increased mean circulatory filling pressure
    c. an increased central venous pressure
    d. distended jugular veins
    e. decreased cardiac output *[handwritten: E –]*

8–7. If you gave a blood transfusion to a patient who had recently experienced a severe hemorrhage, you would expect
    a. to expand arterial volume *[handwritten: – negligible effect on CVP]*
    b. to expand venous volume
    c. to decrease central venous pressure *[handwritten: no. ↑]*
    d. to decrease the mean circulatory filling pressure *[handwritten: ↑]*
    e. to reduce cardiac output *[handwritten: ↑]*

8–8. Which of the following would (directly) (by themselves in the absence of any compensatory responses) tend to decrease central venous (cardiac filling) pressure?
 a. increased sympathetic nerve activity to only the heart   ? → $\downarrow$CO $\downarrow$CVP direct → $\downarrow$ CVP
 b. increased parasympathetic nerve activity to only the heart
 c. increased blood volume
 d. decreased total peripheral resistance $\downarrow$ PVP → $\downarrow$ CVP indirect Periphery then Heart
 e. immersion in water up to the waist $\uparrow$ PVP → $\uparrow$ CVP

— Mean Circulatory Filling Pressure Depends on Blood Volume & Peripheral Venous Tone
note. arteriolar tone ~~decreased~~ isn't Sufficient enough to alter

Central Venous pressure Influences

(+) $\uparrow$ Blood Volume
(+) $\uparrow$ Peripheral Venous tone
(+) $\uparrow$ Peripheral Venous Pressure
(+) $\uparrow$ Venous Return
(+) Skeletal Muscle Contraction pump
(+) Respiratory Pump Suction
(−) Standing i.e. Gravity
(−) $\uparrow$ Cardiac Output

Preload = EDV = CVP, decreasing CVP → $\downarrow$ Preload
 − Diuretics $\downarrow$ Blood Volume   ; ACE, ARB, last resort! CCB
 − Vasodilators! Hydralazine; $\downarrow$BP $\downarrow$ Filtration gradient to
        Dilate blood vessels   ; Venous side $\downarrow$ PVP $\downarrow$ Venous Return $\downarrow$CVP
 − Digoxin $\uparrow$ Contractility
        $\uparrow$SV $\uparrow$ CO $\downarrow$ HR
    − Blocks Na^+/K^+ which Reduces Na^+/Ca^{2+} exchanger activity
        $\uparrow Na^+$ inside $\uparrow Ca^{2+}$ inside $\uparrow$ Trop.C & Ca^{2+} binding.

Regulation of Arterial Pressure 9

OBJECTIVES

The student understands the mechanisms involved in the short-term regulation of arterial pressure:

▶ *Identifies the sensory receptors, afferent pathways, central integrating centers, efferent pathways, and effector organs that participate in the arterial baroreceptor reflex.*

▶ *States the location of the arterial baroreceptors and describes their operation.*

▶ *Describes how changes in the afferent input from arterial baroreceptors influence the activity of the sympathetic and parasympathetic preganglionic fibers.*

▶ *Describes how the sympathetic and parasympathetic outputs from the medullary cardiovascular centers change in response to changes in arterial pressure.*

▶ *Diagrams the chain of events that are initiated by the arterial baroreceptor reflex to compensate for a change in arterial pressure.*

▶ *Describes how inputs to the medullary cardiovascular center from cardiopulmonary baroreceptors, arterial and central chemoreceptors, receptors in skeletal muscle, the cerebral cortex, and the hypothalamus influence sympathetic activity, parasympathetic activity, and mean arterial pressure.*

▶ *Describes and indicates the mechanisms involved in the Bezold–Jarisch reflex, the cerebral ischemic response, the Cushing reflex, the alerting reaction, blushing, vasovagal syncope, the dive reflex, and the cardiovascular responses to emotion and pain.*

The student comprehends the key elements of the commonly accepted "renal mean arterial pressure" theory of long-term arterial pressure regulation.

▶ *Describes baroreceptor adaptation.*

▶ *Describes the influence of changes in body fluid volume on arterial pressure and diagrams the steps involved in this process.*

▶ *Indicates the mechanisms whereby altered arterial pressure alters glomerular filtration rate and renal tubular function to influence urinary output.*

▶ *Describes how mean arterial pressure is adjusted in the long term to that which causes fluid output rate to equal fluid intake rate.*

The student recognizes that our current understanding of all the factors that could be involved in the long-term regulation of arterial pressure is incomplete.

▶ *Describes the basic features of the "CNS-MAP set-point" theory of long-term arterial pressure regulation.*

Appropriate systemic arterial pressure is perhaps the single most important requirement for proper operation of the cardiovascular system. Without sufficient arterial pressure, the brain and the heart do not receive adequate blood flow, no matter what adjustments are made in their vascular resistance by local control mechanisms. In contrast, unnecessary demands are placed on the heart by excessive arterial pressure. The elaborate mechanisms that have evolved for regulating this critical cardiovascular variable are discussed in this chapter.

Arterial pressure is continuously monitored by various sensors located within the body. Whenever arterial pressure varies from normal, multiple reflex responses are initiated, which cause the adjustments in cardiac output, and total peripheral resistance needed to return arterial pressure to its normal value. In the short term (seconds), these adjustments are brought about by changes in the activity of the autonomic nerves leading to the heart and peripheral vessels. In the long term (minutes to days), other mechanisms such as changes in cardiac output brought about by changes in blood volume play an increasingly important role in the control of arterial pressure. The short- and long-term regulations of arterial pressure are discussed in this chapter.

SHORT-TERM REGULATION OF ARTERIAL PRESSURE

Arterial Baroreceptor Reflex

The *arterial baroreceptor reflex* is the single most important mechanism providing short-term regulation of arterial pressure. Recall that the usual components of a reflex pathway include sensory receptors, afferent pathways, integrating centers in the central nervous system (CNS), efferent pathways, and effector organs. As shown in Figure 9–1, the efferent pathways of the arterial baroreceptor reflex are the cardiovascular sympathetic and cardiac parasympathetic nerves. The effector organs are the heart and peripheral blood vessels.

EFFERENT PATHWAYS

Previous chapters have discussed the many actions of the sympathetic and parasympathetic nerves leading to the heart and blood vessels. For both systems, *postganglionic fibers*, whose cell bodies are in ganglia outside the CNS, form the terminal link to the heart and vessels. The influences of these postganglionic fibers on key cardiovascular variables are summarized in Figure 9–1.

The activity of the terminal postganglionic fibers of the autonomic nervous system is determined by the activity of *preganglionic fibers* whose cell bodies lie within the CNS. In the sympathetic pathways, the cell bodies of the preganglionic fibers are located within the spinal cord. These preganglionic neurons have spontaneous activity that is modulated by excitatory and inhibitory inputs, which arise from centers in the brainstem and descend in distinct *excitatory* and *inhibitory* spinal pathways. In the parasympathetic system, the cell bodies of the preganglionic fibers are located within the brainstem. Their spontaneous activity is modulated by inputs from adjacent centers in the brainstem.

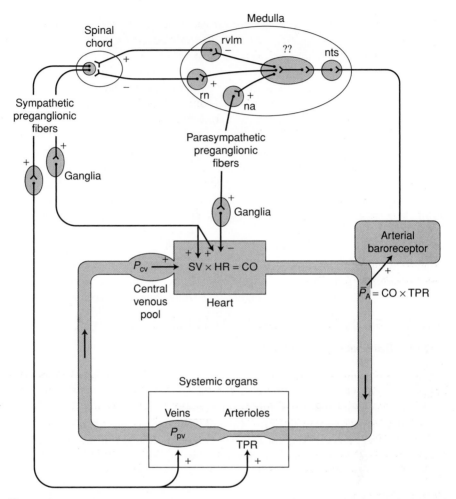

Figure 9-1. Components of the arterial baroreceptor reflex pathway. nts, nucleus tractus solitarius; rvlm, rostral ventrolateral medullary group; rn, raphé nucleus; na, nucleus ambiguus; ??, incompletely mapped integration pathways that may also involve structures outside the medulla.

AFFERENT PATHWAYS

Sensory receptors, called *arterial baroreceptors*, are found in abundance in the walls of the aorta and carotid arteries. Major concentrations of these receptors are found near the arch of the aorta (the *aortic baroreceptors*) and at the bifurcation of the common carotid artery into the internal and external carotid arteries on either side of the neck (the *carotid sinus baroreceptors*). The receptors themselves are mechanoreceptors that sense arterial pressure indirectly from the degree of stretch of the elastic arterial walls. In general, *increased stretch causes an increased action potential generation rate by the arterial baroreceptors.* Baroreceptors actually sense not only absolute stretch

Figure 9–2. The effect of mean arterial pressure on baroreceptor nerve activity.

but also the rate of change of stretch. For this reason, both the mean arterial pressure and the arterial pulse pressure affect baroreceptor firing rate as indicated in Figure 9–2. The dashed curve in Figure 9–2 shows how baroreceptor firing rate is affected by different levels of a steady arterial pressure. The solid curve in Figure 9–2 indicates how baroreceptor firing rate is affected by the mean value of a pulsatile arterial pressure. Note that the presence of pulsations (that of course are normal) increases the baroreceptor firing rate at any given level of mean arterial pressure. Note also that changes in mean arterial pressure near the normal value of 100 mmHg produce the largest changes in baroreceptor discharge rate.

If arterial pressure remains elevated over a period of several days for some reason, the arterial baroreceptor firing rate will gradually return toward normal. Thus, arterial baroreceptors are said to *adapt* to long-term changes in arterial pressure. For this reason, the arterial baroreceptor reflex cannot serve as a mechanism for the long-term regulation of arterial pressure.

Action potentials generated by the carotid sinus baroreceptors travel through the carotid sinus nerves (Hering's nerves), which join with the glossopharyngeal nerves (IX cranial nerves) before entering the CNS. Afferent fibers from the aortic barore-ceptors run to the CNS in the vagus nerves (X cranial nerves). (The vagus nerves contain both afferent and efferent fibers, including, for example, the parasympa-thetic efferent fibers to the heart.)

CENTRAL INTEGRATION

Much of the central integration involved in reflex regulation of the cardiovascular system occurs in the medulla oblongata in what are traditionally referred to as the *medullary cardiovascular centers*. The neural interconnections between the diffuse structures in this area are complex and not completely mapped. Moreover, these structures appear to serve multiple functions including respiratory control, for ex-ample. What is known with a fair degree of certainty is where the cardiovascular afferent and efferent pathways enter and leave the medulla. For example, as indi-cated in Figure 9–1, the afferent sensory information from the arterial baroreceptors enters the medullary *nucleus tractus solitarius,* where it is relayed via polysynaptic pathways to other structures in the medulla (and higher brain centers, such as the hypothalamus, as well). The cell bodies of the efferent vagal parasympathetic cardiac nerves are located primarily in the medullary *nucleus ambiguus.* The sympathetic autonomic efferent information leaves the medulla predominantly from the *rostral ventrolateral medulla* group of neurons (via an excitatory spinal pathway) or the *raphé nucleus* (via an inhibitory spinal pathway). The intermediate processes involved in the actual integration of the sensory information into appropriate sympathetic and parasympathetic responses are not well understood at present. Although much of this integration takes place within the medulla, higher centers such as the hypothalamus are probably involved as well. In this context, knowing the details of the integration process is not as important as appreciating the overall effects that changes in arterial baroreceptor activity have on the activities of parasympathetic and sympathetic cardiovascular nerves.

Several functionally important points about the central control of the autonomic cardiovascular nerves are illustrated in Figure 9–1. The major external influence on the cardiovascular centers comes from the arterial baroreceptors. Because the arterial baroreceptors are active at normal arterial pressures, they supply a tonic input to the central integration centers.

 As indicated in Figure 9–1, the integration process is such that increased input from the arterial baroreceptors tends to simultaneously (1) inhibit the activity of the spinal sympathetic excitatory tract, (2) stimulate the activity of the spinal sympathetic inhibitory tract, and (3) stimulate the activity of parasympathetic preganglionic nerves. Thus, an increase in the arterial baroreceptor discharge rate (caused by increased arterial pressure) causes a decrease in the tonic activity of cardiovascular sympathetic nerves and a simultaneous increase in the tonic activity of cardiac parasympathetic nerves. Conversely, decreased arterial pressure causes increased sympathetic and decreased parasympathetic activity.

OPERATION OF THE ARTERIAL BARORECEPTOR REFLEX

The arterial baroreceptor reflex is a continuously operating control system that automatically makes adjustments to prevent disturbances on the heart and/or vessels from causing large changes in mean arterial pressure. The arterial baroreceptor reflex mechanism acts to regulate arterial pressure in a *negative feedback* manner that is analogous in many ways to the manner in which a thermostatically controlled home heating system operates to regulate inside temperature despite disturbances such as changes in the weather or open windows.[1]

 Figure 9–3 shows many events in the arterial baroreceptor reflex pathway that occur in response to a disturbance of decreased mean arterial pressure.

---

[1] In this analogy, arterial pressure is likened to temperature; the heart is the generator of pressure as the furnace is the generator of heat; dilated arterioles dissipate arterial pressure like open windows lose heat; the arterial baroreceptors monitor arterial pressure as the sensor of a thermostat monitors temperature; and the electronics of the thermostat control the furnace as the medullary cardiovascular centers regulate the operation of the heart. Because home thermostats do not usually also regulate the operation of the windows, there is no analogy to the reflex medullary control of arterioles. The pressure that the arterial baroreflex strives to maintain is analogous to the temperature setting on the thermostat dial.

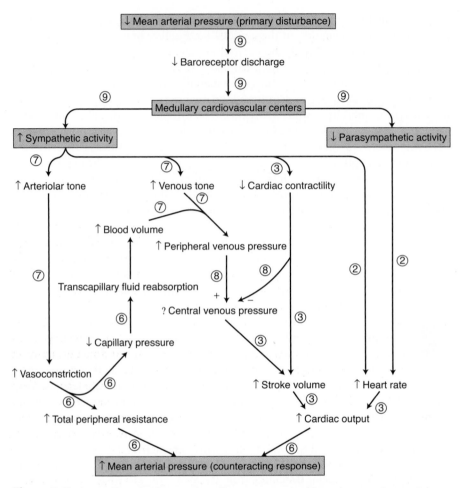

Figure 9–3. Immediate cardiovascular adjustments caused by a decrease in arterial blood pressure. Circled numbers indicate the chapter in which each interaction is discussed.

All the events shown in Figure 9–3 have already been discussed, and each should be carefully examined (and reviewed if necessary) at this point because a great many of the interactions that are essential to understanding cardiovascular physiology are summarized in this figure.

Note that in Figure 9–3 the overall response of the arterial baroreceptor reflex to the disturbance of decreased mean arterial pressure is increased mean arterial pressure (ie, the response tends to counteract the disturbance). A disturbance of increased mean arterial pressure would elicit events exactly opposite to those shown in Figure 9–3 and produce the response of decreased mean arterial pressure; again, the response tends to counteract the disturbance. The homeostatic benefits of the reflex action should be apparent.

One should recall that nervous control of vessels is more important in some areas such as the kidney, the skin, and the splanchnic organs than in the brain and the heart muscle. Thus, the reflex response to a fall in arterial pressure may, for example, include a significant increase in renal vascular resistance and a decrease in renal blood flow without changing the cerebral vascular resistance or blood flow. The peripheral vascular adjustments associated with the arterial baroreceptor reflex take place primarily in organs with strong sympathetic vascular control.

Other Cardiovascular Reflexes and Responses

Seemingly in spite of the arterial baroreceptor reflex mechanism, large and rapid changes in mean arterial pressure occur in certain physiological and pathological situations. These reactions are caused by influences on the medullary cardiovascular centers *other* than those from the arterial baroreceptors. As outlined in the following sections, these inputs on the medullary cardiovascular centers arise from many types of peripheral and central receptors as well as from "higher centers" in the CNS such as the hypothalamus and the cortex.

The analogy was made earlier that the arterial baroreceptor reflex operates to control arterial pressure somewhat as a home heating system acts to control inside temperature. Such a system automatically acts to counteract changes in temperature caused by such things as an open window or a dirty furnace. It does not, however, resist changes in temperature caused by someone's resetting of the thermostat dial—in fact, the basic temperature-regulating mechanisms cooperate wholeheartedly in adjusting the temperature to the new desired value. The temperature setting on a home thermostat's dial has a useful conceptual analogy in cardiovascular physiology often referred to as the "*set point*" for arterial pressure. *Most (but not all) of the influences that are about to be discussed influence arterial pressure as if they changed the arterial baroreceptor reflex's set point for pressure regulation.* Consequently, the arterial baroreceptor reflex does not resist most of these pressure disturbances, but actually assists in producing them.

REFLEXES FROM RECEPTORS IN THE HEART AND LUNGS

A host of mechanoreceptors and chemoreceptors that can elicit reflex cardiovascular responses have been identified in the atria, ventricles, coronary vessels, and lungs. The role of these *cardiopulmonary receptors* in the neurohumoral control of the cardiovascular system is, in most cases, incompletely understood, but evidence is accumulating that they may be involved significantly in many physiological and pathological states.

One general function that the cardiopulmonary receptors perform is sensing the pressure (or volume) in the atria and central venous pool. Increased central venous pressure and volume cause receptor activation by stretch, which elicits a reflex decrease in sympathetic activity. Decreased central venous pressure produces the opposite response. Whatever the details, it is clear that cardiopulmonary baroreflexes normally exert a tonic inhibitory influence on sympathetic activity and play an arguably important, but not yet completely defined, role in normal cardiovascular regulation.[2]

CHEMORECEPTOR REFLEXES

Low P_{O_2} and/or high P_{CO_2} levels in the arterial blood cause reflex increases in respiratory rate *and* mean arterial pressure. These responses appear to be a result of increased activity of *arterial chemoreceptors*, located in the carotid arteries and the arch of the aorta, and *central chemoreceptors*, located somewhere within the CNS. Chemoreceptors probably play little role in the normal regulation of arterial pressure because arterial blood P_{O_2} and P_{CO_2} are normally held very nearly constant by respiratory control mechanisms.

An extremely strong reaction called the *cerebral ischemic response* is triggered by inadequate brain blood flow (ischemia) and can produce a more intense sympathetic vasoconstriction and cardiac stimulation than is elicited by any other influence on the cardiovascular control centers. Presumably the cerebral ischemic response is initiated by chemoreceptors located within the CNS. However, if cerebral blood flow is severely inadequate for several minutes, the cerebral ischemic response wanes and is replaced by marked loss of sympathetic activity. Presumably this situation results when function of the nerve cells in the cardiovascular centers becomes directly depressed by the unfavorable chemical conditions in the cerebrospinal fluid.

Whenever intracranial pressure is increased—for example, by tumor growth or trauma-induced bleeding within the rigid cranium—there is a parallel rise in arterial pressure. This is called the *Cushing reflex.* It can cause mean arterial pressures of more than 200 mmHg in severe cases of intracranial pressure elevation. The obvious benefit of the Cushing reflex is that it prevents collapse of cranial vessels and thus preserves adequate brain blood flow in the face of large increases in intracranial pressure. The mechanisms responsible for the Cushing reflex are not known but could involve the central chemoreceptors. A hallmark of the Cushing reflex is acutely increased arterial pressure in spite of accompanying bradycardia. It seems as if the short-term arterial baroreceptor reflex is attempting to fight this disturbance.

REFLEXES FROM RECEPTORS IN EXERCISING SKELETAL MUSCLE

Reflex tachycardia and increased arterial pressure can be elicited by stimulation of certain afferent fibers from the skeletal muscle. These pathways may be activated by chemoreceptors responding to muscle ischemia, which occurs with strong, sustained static (isometric) exercise. This input may contribute to the marked increase in blood pressure that accompanies such isometric efforts. It is uncertain as to what extent this reflex contributes to the cardiovascular responses to dynamic (rhythmic) muscle exercise.

---

[2] Certain other reflexes originating from receptors in the cardiopulmonary region have been described that may be important in specific pathological situations. For example, the *Bezold–Jarisch* reflex that involves marked bradycardia and hypotension is elicited by application of strong stimuli to coronary vessel (or myocardial) chemoreceptors concentrated primarily in the posterior wall of the left ventricle. Activation of this reflex causes certain myocardial infarction patients to present with bradycardia instead of the expected tachycardia.

THE DIVE REFLEX

Aquatic animals respond to diving with a remarkable bradycardia and intense vasoconstriction in all systemic organs except the brain and the heart. The response serves to allow prolonged submersion by limiting the rate of oxygen use and by directing blood flow to essential organs. A similar but less dramatic dive reflex can be elicited in humans by simply immersing the face in water. (Cold water enhances the response.) The response involves the unusual combination of bradycardia produced by enhanced cardiac parasympathetic activity and peripheral vasoconstriction caused by enhanced sympathetic activity that is a rare exception to the general rule that sympathetic and parasympathetic nerves are activated in reciprocal fashion. The dive reflex is sometimes used clinically to reflexly activate cardiac parasympathetic nerves for the purpose of interrupting atrial tachyarrhythmias.

Another, but unrelated, clinical technique for activating parasympathetic nerves in an attempt to interrupt atrial tachyarrhythmias is called *carotid massage*. In essence, massage of the neck is done to cause physical deformation of the carotid sinuses and "trick" them into sending a "high-pressure" alarm to the medullary control centers.

CARDIOVASCULAR RESPONSES ASSOCIATED WITH EMOTION

Cardiovascular responses are frequently associated with certain states of emotion. These responses originate in the cerebral cortex and reach the medullary cardiovascular centers through corticohypothalamic pathways. The least complicated of these responses is the *blushing* that is often detectable in individuals with lightly pigmented skin during states of embarrassment. The blushing response involves a loss of sympathetic vasoconstrictor activity *only* to particular cutaneous vessels, and this produces the blushing by allowing engorgement of the cutaneous venous sinuses.

Excitement or a sense of danger often elicits a complex behavioral pattern called the *alerting reaction* (also called the "defense" or "fight or flight" response). The alerting reaction involves a host of responses such as pupillary dilation and increased skeletal muscle tenseness that are generally appropriate preparations for some form of intense physical activity. The cardiovascular component of the alerting reaction is an increase in blood pressure caused by a general increase in cardiovascular sympathetic nervous activity and a decrease in cardiac parasympathetic activity. Centers in the *posterior hypothalamus* are presumed to be involved in the alerting reaction because many of the components of this multifaceted response can be experimentally reproduced by electrical stimulation of this area. The general cardiovascular effects are mediated via hypothalamic communications with the medullary cardiovascular centers.

Some individuals respond to situations of extreme stress by fainting, a situation referred to clinically as *vasovagal syncope*. The loss of consciousness is due to decreased cerebral blood flow that is itself produced by a sudden dramatic loss of arterial blood pressure that, in turn, occurs as a result of a sudden loss of sympathetic tone and a simultaneous large increase in parasympathetic tone and decrease in the heart rate. The influences on the medullary cardiovascular centers that produce vasovagal syncope appear to come from the cortex via depressor centers in the *anterior hypothalamus.* It has been suggested that vasovagal syncope is analogous to the "playing dead" response to peril used by some animals. Fortunately, unconsciousness (combined with becoming horizontal) seems to quickly remove this serious disturbance to the normal mechanisms of arterial pressure control in humans.

The extent to which cardiovascular variables, in particular blood pressure, are normally affected by an emotional state is currently a topic of extreme interest and considerable research. As yet the answer is unclear. However, the therapeutic value of being able, for example, to learn to consciously reduce one's blood pressure would be incalculable.

CENTRAL COMMAND

The term *central command* is used to imply an input from the cerebral cortex to lower brain centers during voluntary muscle exercise. The concept is that the same cortical drives that initiate somatomotor (skeletal muscle) activity also simultaneously initiate cardiovascular (and respiratory) adjustments appropriate to support that activity. In the absence of any other obvious causes, central command is at present the best explanation as to why both mean arterial pressure and respiration increase during voluntary exercise.

REFLEX RESPONSES TO PAIN

Pain can have either a positive or negative influence on arterial pressure. Generally, superficial or cutaneous pain causes a rise in blood pressure in a manner similar to that associated with the alerting response and perhaps over many of the same pathways. Deep pain from receptors in the viscera or joints, however, often causes a cardiovascular response similar to that which accompanies vasovagal syncope, that is, decreased sympathetic tone, increased parasympathetic tone, and a serious decrease in blood pressure. This response may contribute to the state of shock that often accompanies crushing injuries and/or joint displacement.

TEMPERATURE REGULATION REFLEXES

Certain special cardiovascular reflexes that involve the control of skin blood flow have evolved as part of the body temperature regulation mechanisms. Temperature regulation responses are controlled primarily by the hypothalamus, which can operate through the cardiovascular centers to discretely control the sympathetic activity to cutaneous vessels and thus skin blood flow. The sympathetic activity to cutaneous vessels is extremely responsive to changes in hypothalamic temperature. Measurable changes in cutaneous blood flow result from changes in hypothalamic temperature of tenths of a degree Celsius.

Cutaneous vessels are influenced by reflexes involved in both arterial pressure regulation and temperature regulation. When the appropriate cutaneous vascular responses for temperature regulation and pressure regulation are contradictory, as they are, for example, during strenuous exercise in a hot environment, then the temperature-regulating influences on cutaneous blood vessels usually prevail.

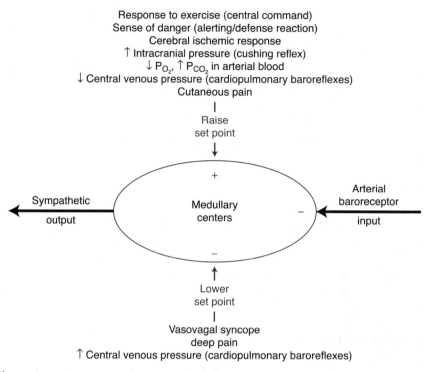

Response to exercise (central command)
Sense of danger (alerting/defense reaction)
Cerebral ischemic response
↑ Intracranial pressure (cushing reflex)
↓ P_{O_2}, ↑ P_{CO_2} in arterial blood
↓ Central venous pressure (cardiopulmonary baroreflexes)
Cutaneous pain

Raise
set point

+

Sympathetic
output

Medullary
centers

−

Arterial
baroreceptor
input

−

Lower
set point

Vasovagal syncope
deep pain
↑ Central venous pressure (cardiopulmonary baroreflexes)

Figure 9–4. Summary of the factors that influence the set point of the arterial baroreceptor reflex.

SUMMARY

Most of the influences on the medullary cardiovascular centers that have been discussed in the preceding sections are summarized in Figure 9–4. This figure is intended first to reemphasize that the arterial baroreceptors normally and continually supply the major input to the medullary centers. The arterial baroreceptor input is shown as inhibitory because an increase in arterial baroreceptor firing rate results in a decrease in sympathetic output. (Decreased sympathetic output should be taken to imply also a simultaneous increase in parasympathetic output that is not shown in this figure.)

As is indicated in Figure 9–4, the *nonarterial baroreceptor influences* on the medullary cardiovascular centers fall into two categories: (1) those that *increase* arterial pressure by raising the set point for the arterial baroreceptor reflex and thus cause an increase in sympathetic activity and (2) those that *decrease* arterial pressure by lowering the set point for the arterial baroreceptor reflex and thus cause a decrease in sympathetic activity. Note that certain responses that have been discussed are not included in Figure 9–4. The complex combination of stimuli involved in the dive reflex causes simultaneous sympathetic and parasympathetic activation and cannot be simply classified as either pressure raising or pressure lowering. Also, temperature stimuli that discretely affect cutaneous vessels but not general cardiovascular sympathetic and parasympathetic activity have not been included in Figure 9–4.

The nonarterial baroreceptor influences shown in Figure 9–4 may be viewed as disturbances on the cardiovascular system that act on the medullary cardiovascular centers as opposed to disturbances that act on the heart and vessels. These disturbances cause sympathetic activity and arterial pressure to change in the *same direction*. Recall from the discussion of the arterial baroreceptor reflex that cardiovascular disturbances that act on the heart or vessels (such as blood loss or heart failure) produce *reciprocal* changes in arterial pressure and sympathetic activity. These facts are often useful in the clinical diagnoses of blood pressure abnormalities. For example, patients commonly present in the physician's office with high blood pressure in combination with elevated heart rate (implying elevated sympathetic activity). These same-direction changes in arterial pressure and sympathetic activity suggest that the problem lies not in the periphery but rather with an abnormal pressure-raising input to the medullary cardiovascular centers. The physician should immediately think of those set-point raising influences listed in the top half of Figure 9–4 that would simultaneously raise sympathetic activity and arterial pressure. Often, such a patient does not have chronic hypertension but rather is just experiencing a temporary blood pressure elevation due to the anxiety of undergoing a physical examination.

A more rigorous analysis of the operation of the arterial baroreflex is presented in Appendix E. It is not essential reading but the serious students may find it enlightening.

LONG-TERM REGULATION OF ARTERIAL PRESSURE

Long-term regulation of arterial pressure is a topic of extreme clinical relevance because of the prevalence of *hypertension* (sustained excessive arterial blood pressure) in our society. The most long-standing and generally accepted theory of long-term pressure regulation is that it crucially involves the kidneys, their sodium handling, and ultimately the regulation of blood volume. This theory is sometimes referred to as the "renal-MAP set-point" or "fluid balance" model of long-term arterial blood pressure control. In essence, this theory asserts that in the long term, mean arterial pressure is whatever it needs to be to maintain an appropriate blood volume through arterial pressure's direct effects on renal function. At the end of this chapter, we present some alternative hypotheses that argue that the generally accepted "renal-MAP" model of long-term pressure regulation is overly simplistic and incomplete.

Fluid Balance and Arterial Pressure

Several key factors in the long-term regulation of arterial blood pressure have already been considered. First is the fact that the baroreceptor reflex, however well it counteracts temporary disturbances in arterial pressure, cannot effectively regulate arterial pressure in the long term for the simple reason that the baroreceptor firing rate adapts to prolonged changes in arterial pressure.

The second pertinent fact is that circulating blood volume can influence arterial pressure because:

↓ Blood volume
↓
↓ Peripheral venous pressure
↓
Left shift of venous function curve
↓
↓ Central venous pressure
↓
↓ Cardiac output
↓
↓ Arterial pressure

A fact yet to be considered is that arterial pressure has a profound influence on urinary output rate and thus affects total body fluid volume. Because blood volume is one of the components of the total body fluid, blood volume alterations accompany changes in total body fluid volume. The mechanisms are such that an *increase in arterial pressure* causes an increase in urinary output rate and thus a *decrease in blood volume.* But, as outlined in the preceding sequence, decreased blood volume tends to lower arterial pressure. Thus, the complete sequence of events that are initiated by an increase in arterial pressure can be listed as follows:

↑ Arterial pressure (disturbance)
↓
↑ Urinary output rate
↓
↓ Fluid volume
↓
↓ Blood volume
↓
↓ Cardiac output
↓
↓ Arterial pressure (compensation)

Note the negative feedback nature of this sequence of events: increased arterial pressure leads to fluid volume depletion, which tends to lower arterial pressure. Conversely, an initial disturbance of decreased arterial pressure would lead to fluid volume expansion, which would tend to increase arterial pressure. Because of negative feedback, these events constitute a *fluid volume mechanism* for regulating arterial pressure.

As indicated in Figure 9–5, both the arterial baroreceptor reflex and this fluid volume mechanism are negative feedback loops that regulate arterial pressure. Although the arterial baroreceptor reflex is very quick to counteract disturbances in arterial pressure, hours or even days may be required before a change in urinary output rate produces a significant accumulation or loss of total body fluid volume. Whatever this fluid volume mechanism lacks in speed, however, it more than makes

Figure 9–5. Mechanisms of short- and long-term regulations of arterial pressure. TPR, total peripheral resistance; CO, cardiac output.

up for in persistence. As long as there is any inequality between the fluid intake rate and the urinary output rate, fluid volume is changing and this fluid volume mechanism has not completed its adjustment of arterial pressure. The fluid volume mechanism is in equilibrium only when the urinary output rate exactly equals the fluid intake rate.[3] *In the long term, the arterial pressure can only be that which makes the urinary output rate equal to the fluid intake rate.*

The baroreceptor reflex is, of course, essential for counteracting rapid changes in arterial pressure. The fluid volume mechanism, however, determines the long-term level of arterial pressure because it slowly overwhelms all other influences. Through adaptation, the baroreceptor mechanism adjusts itself so that it operates to prevent acute changes in blood pressure from the prevailing long-term level as determined through fluid balance.

---

[3] In the present discussion, assume that fluid intake rate represents that in excess of the obligatory fluid losses that normally occur in the feces and by transpiration from the skin and structures in the respiratory tract. The processes that regulate voluntary fluid intake (thirst) are not well understood but seem to involve many of the same factors that influence urinary output (eg, blood volume and osmolality). Angiotensin II may be an important factor in the regulation of thirst.

Effect of Arterial Pressure on Urinary Output Rate

A key element in the fluid balance mechanism of arterial pressure regulation is the effect that arterial pressure has on the renal urine production rate. The mechanisms responsible for this are briefly described here with emphasis on their cardiovascular implications.

As indicated in Chapter 1, the kidneys play a major role in homeostasis by regulating the electrolyte composition of the plasma and thus the entire internal environment. One of the major plasma electrolytes regulated by the kidneys is the sodium ion. To regulate the electrolyte composition, a large fraction of the plasma fluid that flows into the kidneys is filtered across the *glomerular capillaries* so that it enters the *renal tubules*. The fluid that passes from the blood into the renal tubules is called the *glomerular filtrate*, and the rate at which this process occurs is called the *glomerular filtration rate*. Glomerular filtration is a transcapillary fluid movement whose rate is influenced by hydrostatic and oncotic pressures as indicated in Chapter 6. The primary cause of continual glomerular filtration is that glomerular capillary hydrostatic pressure is normally very high ($\simeq 60$ mmHg). The glomerular filtration rate is decreased by factors that decrease glomerular capillary pressure, for example, decreased arterial blood pressure or vasoconstriction of preglomerular renal arterioles.

Once fluid is filtered into the renal tubules, it either (1) is *reabsorbed* and reenters the cardiovascular system or (2) is passed along renal tubules and eventually *excreted* as urine. Thus, urine production is the net result of glomerular filtration and renal tubular fluid reabsorption:

Urinary output rate = glomerular filtration rate − renal fluid reabsorption rate

Actually, most of the reabsorption of fluid that has entered renal tubules as glomerular filtrate occurs because sodium is actively pumped out of the tubules by cells in the tubular wall. When sodium leaves the tubules, osmotic forces are produced that cause water to leave with it. Thus, any factor that promotes renal tubular sodium reabsorption (sodium retention) tends to increase the renal fluid reabsorption rate and consequently decrease the urinary output rate. The blood concentration of the hormone *aldosterone*, which is produced by the adrenal glands, is the primary regulator of the rate of sodium reabsorption by renal tubular cells. Adrenal release of aldosterone is, in turn, regulated largely by the circulating level of another hormone, *angiotensin II*, whose plasma concentration is determined by the plasma concentration of *renin*, an enzyme that is produced in the kidneys. Renin actually catalyzes the formation of an inactive decapeptide, *angiotensin I*, from *angiotensinogen*, a circulating precursor protein. Angiotensin I then gets quickly converted to angiotensin II (an octapeptide) by the action of *angiotensin-converting enzyme* that is located on the surface of endothelial cells. The combination of elements involved in this whole sequence of events is referred to as the *renin–angiotensin–aldosterone system.*

The rate of renin release by the kidneys is influenced by several factors. An increase in the activity of renal sympathetic nerves causes a direct release of renin through a β_1-adrenergic mechanism. Also, renin release is triggered by factors associated with a lowered glomerular filtration rate. The activation of sympathetic vasoconstrictor nerves to renal arterioles thus indirectly causes renin release via lowered glomerular capillary hydrostatic pressure and glomerular filtration rate. The important fact to keep in mind, from a cardiovascular standpoint, is that anything that causes renin release causes a decrease in urinary output rate because increased renin causes increased sodium (and therefore fluid) reabsorption from renal tubules.[4]

Urinary output rate is also influenced by vasopressin (antidiuretic hormone) released from the posterior pituitary. Vasopressin regulates the permeability of certain portions of the kidney tubule in such a way that when the blood levels of the hormone are elevated, water is reabsorbed from the tubule and the kidney produces only small volumes of highly concentrated urine. The production of vasopressin in the hypothalamus and its release from the pituitary are stimulated by many factors including increased extracellular fluid osmolality, decreased input from cardiopulmonary baroreceptors, and decreased input from arterial baroreceptors. In the case of the latter two influences on vasopressin release, the overall result is to decrease urinary output rate whenever arterial pressure and/or central blood volume is below normal.

Some major mechanisms that lead to decreased urinary output rate are summarized in Figure 9–6. Most important, this figure shows that urinary output rate is linked to arterial pressure by many synergistic pathways. Because of this, modest changes in arterial pressure are associated with large changes in urinary output rate.

The observed relation between arterial pressure and urinary output for a healthy person is shown in Figure 9–7. Recall that, in the steady state, the urinary output rate must always equal the fluid intake rate and that changes in fluid volume will automatically adjust arterial pressure until this is so. Thus, a healthy person with a normal fluid intake rate will have, as a long-term average, the arterial pressure associated with point A in Figure 9–7. Because of the steepness of the curve shown in Figure 9–7, even rather marked changes in fluid intake rate have minor influences on the arterial pressure of a healthy individual.

Role of the CNS in Long-Term Arterial Pressure Regulation

Many argue that the CNS plays a more important role in the long-term regulation of arterial pressure than is implied by the foregoing "renal fluid balance" model. The crux of the dispute is whether the kidney or the brain is the ultimate controller of long-term blood pressure. In particular, the CNS proponents argue that there is a

---

[4] Although the renin–angiotensin–aldosterone system is clearly the primary mechanism for the regulation of renal tubular sodium reabsorption, many believe that other factors are involved. A polypeptide natriuretic (salt-losing) factor has been identified in granules of cardiac atrial cells. Atrial distention causes the release of this *atrial natriuretic peptide* into the blood. The possibility that the heart itself may serve as an endocrine organ in the regulation of body fluid volume is stimulating much research interest.

Figure 9–6. Mechanisms by which arterial pressure influences urinary output rate.

Figure 9–7. The effect of arterial pressure on urinary output rate in a healthy person.

"CNS arterial pressure set point" designed to maintain proper cerebral blood flow and function as opposed to a "renal arterial pressure set point" designed to maintain proper blood volume.

Indeed, even the short-term regulation of arterial pressure is a complex issue that involves many inputs to the medullary cardiovascular control centers in addition to that from the arterial baroreceptors (see Fig. 9–4). It is largely unknown to what extents these "other" influences might be involved in long-term pressure regulation as well. Moreover, the Cushing reflex described earlier clearly indicates the existence of a powerful pressure-regulating mechanism aimed at maintaining adequate brain blood flow.

We remind the student that, whatever the purpose of long-term arterial pressure regulation, changes in mean arterial pressure can be accomplished only by changing cardiac output and/or total peripheral resistance. Blood volume is undeniably one important determinant of cardiac output. Thus, we (the authors of this text) conclude that there are elements of truth in both the renal and CNS theories of long-term blood pressure control. Hopefully, this debate will ultimately result in some melding of the theories that will improve our understanding of what factors cause chronic hypertension.

KEY CONCEPTS

 Arterial pressure is closely regulated to ensure adequate blood flow to the tissues.

 The arterial baroreceptor reflex is responsible for regulating arterial pressure in the short term on a second-to-second and moment-to-moment basis.

 The arterial baroreceptor reflex involves the following: pressure sensing by stretch-sensitive baroreceptor nerve endings in the walls of arteries; neural integrating centers in the brainstem that adjust autonomic nerve activity in response to the pressure information they receive from the arterial baroreceptors; and responses of the heart and vessels to changes in autonomic nerve activity.

 Overall, the arterial baroreflex operates such that increases in arterial pressure lead to an essentially immediate decrease in sympathetic nerve activity and a simultaneous increase in parasympathetic nerve activity (and vice versa).

 The brainstem integrating centers also receive nonarterial baroreceptor inputs that can raise or lower the set point for short-term arterial pressure regulation.

 In the long term, arterial pressure is regulated by changes in blood volume that come about because arterial pressure has a strong influence on urinary output rate by the kidney.

? STUDY QUESTIONS

9–1. Consider the various components of the arterial baroreceptor reflex and predict whether the following variables will increase or decrease in response to a rise in arterial pressure.

a. arterial baroreceptor firing rate

b. parasympathetic activity to the heart

c. sympathetic activity to the heart

d. arteriolar tone

e. venous tone

f. peripheral venous pressure

g. total peripheral resistance

h. cardiac output

9–2. Massage of the neck over the carotid sinus area in a person experiencing a bout of paroxysmal atrial tachycardia is often effective in terminating the episode. Why?

9–3. Indicate whether mean arterial pressure, after all adjustments, is increased or decreased by the following stimuli:

a. low oxygen in arterial blood

b. increased intracranial pressure

c. increased cardiac filling pressure

d. sense of danger

e. visceral pain

9–4. Describe the immediate direct and reflex cardiovascular consequences of giving a healthy person a drug that blocks α_1-adrenergic receptors.

9–5. What net short-term alterations in mean arterial pressure and sympathetic activity would the following produce?

a. blood loss through hemorrhage

b. cutaneous pain

c. systemic hypoxia

d. local metabolic vasodilation in the skeletal muscle

9–6. Your patient has lower than normal mean arterial pressure and higher than normal pulse rate. Which of the following are possible diagnoses?

a. low blood volume

b. anxiety

c. a cardiac valve problem

d. elevated intracranial pressure

9–7. In the normal operation of the arterial baroreceptor reflex, a cardiovascular disturbance that lowers mean arterial pressure will evoke a decrease in

a. baroreceptor firing rate

b. sympathetic nerve activity

c. the heart rate

d. total peripheral resistance

e. myocardial contractility

9–8. In general, normal kidneys tend to retain sodium and fluid in the body whenever
  a. arterial pressure is high
  b. parasympathetic nerve activity is high
  c. sympathetic nerve activity is high
  d. plasma aldosterone levels are low
  e. plasma renin levels are low

9–9. If your patient's mean systemic arterial pressure changes, it is definitely because of changes in
  a. the heart rate and/or myocardial contractility
  b. cardiac output and/or total peripheral resistance
  c. blood volume and/or venous tone
  d. sympathetic and/or parasympathetic nerve activity
  e. arterial compliance and/or stroke volume

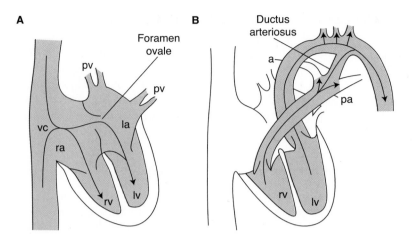

Figure 10–6. Fetal circulation during (**A**) cardiac filling and (**B**) cardiac ejection. pv, pulmonary veins; la, left atrium; lv, left ventricle; rv, right ventricle; ra, right atrium; vc, venae cavae; a, aorta; pa, pulmonary artery.

decrease that on the right. This indirectly causes left atrial pressure to increase above that in the right atrium so that the pressure gradient for flow through the foramen ovale is reversed. Reverse flow through the foramen ovale is, however, prevented by a flap-like valve that covers the opening in the left atrium. Normally, the foramen ovale is eventually closed permanently by the growth of fibrous tissue.

Pediatric Cardiovascular Characteristics

Cardiovascular variables change significantly between birth and adulthood. The healthy neonate has, by adult standards, a high resting heart rate (average of 140 beats per minute) and a low arterial blood pressure (average of 60/35 mmHg). These average values rapidly change over the first year (to 120 beats per minute and 100/65 mmHg, respectively). By the time the child enters adolescence, these values are near adult levels.

Pulmonary vascular resistance decreases precipitously at birth as described earlier and then continues to decline during the first year, at which time pulmonary pressures resemble adult levels. These resistance changes appear to be due to a progressive remodeling of the microvascular arterioles from thick-walled, small-diameter vessels to thin-walled, large-diameter microvessels.

It is noteworthy that distinct differences between right and left ventricular mass and wall thickness develop only after birth. Presumably they arise because of a hypertrophic response of the left ventricle to the increased afterload it must assume at birth. Accordingly, the electrocardiogram of children shows an early right ventricular dominance (electrical axis orientation) that converts to the normal left ventricular dominance during childhood.

Heart murmurs are also quite common in childhood and have been reported to be present in as many as 50% of healthy children. Most of these murmurs fall in the category of "innocent" murmurs, resulting from normal cardiac tissue vibrations, high flow through valves, and thin chest walls that make noises from the vasculature easy to hear. Less than 1% of them result from various congenital heart defects.

Growth and development of the vascular system parallels growth and development of the body with most of the local and reflex regulatory mechanisms operational shortly after birth.

Cardiovascular Changes with Normal Aging

In general, as persons get older, they get slower, stiffer, and drier. Connective tissue becomes less elastic, capillary density decreases in many tissues, mitotic activity of dividing cells becomes slower, and fixed postmitotic cells (such as nerve and muscle fibers) are lost. Although these changes do not, in general, alter the basic physiological processes, they do have an influence on the rate at which various homeostatic mechanisms operate.

Age-dependent changes that occur in the heart include (1) a decrease in the resting and maximum cardiac index, (2) a decrease in the maximum heart rate, (3) an increase in the contraction and relaxation time of the heart muscle, (4) an increase in the myocardial stiffness during diastole, (5) a decrease in the number of functioning myocytes, and (6) an accumulation of pigment in the myocardial cells.

Changes that occur in the vascular bed with age include a decrease in capillary density in some tissues, a decrease in arterial and venous compliance, and an increase in total peripheral vascular resistance. These changes combine to produce the age-dependent increases in arterial pulse pressure and mean arterial pressure that are discussed in Chapter 6 (see Figure 6–10). The increases in arterial pressure impose a greater afterload on the heart, which may be partially responsible for the age-dependent decreases in cardiac index.

Arterial baroreceptor-induced responses to changes in blood pressure are blunted with age. This is due in part to a decrease in afferent activity from the arterial baroreceptors because of the age-dependent increase in arterial rigidity. In addition, the total amount of norepinephrine contained in the sympathetic nerve endings of the myocardium decreases with age, and the myocardial responsiveness to catecholamines declines. Thus, the efferent component of the reflex is also compromised. These changes may partially account for the apparent age-dependent sluggishness in the responses to postural changes and recovery from exercise.

It is important (although often difficult) to separate age-dependent alterations from disease-induced changes in physiological function. Cardiovascular diseases are the major cause of death in an aging population. Atherosclerosis and hypertension are the primary culprits in many populations. These "diseases" lack the universality necessary to be categorized as aging processes but generally occur with increasing incidence in the older population. Pharmacological interventions and reduction of risk factors (smoking, obesity, inactivity, and high-fat or high-sodium diets) by modification of lifestyle can alter the incidence, intensity, and progression of these diseases. It is also possible that some of the previously mentioned interventions may prevent early expression of some of the normal aging processes and prolong the lifespan of a given individual. No practical intervention, however, is currently available that will increase the maximum potential lifespan of humans.

EFFECT OF GENDER

 There are a few well-documented gender-dependent differences in the cardiovascular system. Compared with age-matched men, premenopausal women have a lower left ventricular mass to body mass ratio, which may reflect a lower cardiac afterload in women. This may result from their lower arterial blood pressure, greater aortic compliance, and improved ability to induce vasodilatory mechanisms (such as endothelial-dependent flow-mediated vasodilation). These differences are thought to be related to protective effects of estrogen and may account for the lowered risk of premenopausal women for developing cardiovascular disease. After menopause, these gender differences disappear. In fact, older women with ischemic heart disease often have a worse prognosis than men.

There are also gender-dependent differences in cardiac electrical properties. Women often have lower intrinsic heart rates and longer QT intervals than do men. They are at greater risk of developing long-QT syndrome and torsades de pointes. They are also twice as likely as men to have atrioventricular nodal reentry tachycardias.

However, it should be noted that most basic cardiovascular physiological processes are not greatly influenced by gender and that individual differences in physiological responses within genders are usually as large as, or larger than, differences between genders.

KEY CONCEPTS

 Cardiovascular responses to physiological stresses should be evaluated in terms of the initial effects of the primary disturbance and the subsequent effects of the reflex compensatory responses.

Changes in intrathoracic pressure due to respiratory activity have significant effects on the cardiovascular system, partly by influencing venous return and cardiac filling.

Gravity, and hence body position, has a significant effect on the cardiovascular system, and various reflex compensatory mechanisms are required to overcome peripheral venous pooling and reduced cardiac filling that accompanies the upright position.

 Long-term bed rest causes decreases in circulating blood volume that contributes to orthostatic hypotension.

The primary cardiovascular disturbances of exercise (central command and muscle vasodilation) evoke immediate reflex compensatory activity, which permits major changes in muscle blood flow and cardiac output.

Chronic exercise (training) evokes compensatory adjustments in blood volume, cardiovascular characteristics and muscle metabolic processes, permitting greater exercise efficiency.

Pregnancy-induced cardiovascular changes, including a major decrease in total peripheral resistance due to the developing placenta, evoke a significant increase in circulating maternal blood volume.

Circulatory pathways in the fetus are significantly different from those of the newborn and change abruptly at birth with the first breath.

Pediatric cardiovascular characteristics (high resting heart rates and low arterial blood pressures) gradually change to reach the normal adult levels during early adolescence.

Aging results in decreases in the maximal capabilities of cardiovascular responses that are distinct from any disease processes.

Gender influences several cardiovascular characteristics and disease susceptibility particularly before the age of menopause in women.

STUDY QUESTIONS

10–1. How are the thin-walled capillaries in the feet able to withstand pressures greater than 100 mmHg in a standing individual without rupturing?

10–2. Soldiers faint when standing at attention on a very hot day more often than on a cooler day. Why?

10–3. For several days after an extended period of bed rest, patients often become dizzy when they stand upright quickly because of an exaggerated transient fall in arterial pressure (orthostatic hypotension). Why might this be so?

10–4. Vertical immersion to the neck in tepid water produces a diuresis in many individuals. What mechanisms might account for this phenomenon?

10–5. How is the decrease in skeletal muscle vascular resistance evident from the data presented in Figure 10–4?

10–6. Is a decrease in total peripheral resistance implied in Figure 10–4?

10–7. What in Figure 10–4 implies increased sympathetic activity?

10–8. From the information given in Figure 10–4,

    a. Calculate the resting and exercising stroke volumes (SVs).

    b. Calculate the resting and exercising end-diastolic volumes (EDVs).

    c. Calculate the resting and exercising end-systolic volumes (ESVs).

    d. Construct a sketch that indicates, as accurately as possible, how this exercise affects the left ventricular volume–pressure cycle.

10–9. The "iron lung," used to help polio victims breathe in the mid-20th century, applied an external intermittent negative pressure to the patient's thoracic cavity. How is this better than positive-pressure ventilation of the patient's lungs?

10–10. Blood pressure can rise to extremely high levels during strenuous isometric exercise maneuvers like weight lifting. Why?

10–11. All the following tend to occur when a person lies down. Which one is the primary disturbance that causes all the others to happen?

    a. The heart rate will decrease.

    b. Stroke volume will increase.

    c. Sympathetic activity will decrease.

    d. Parasympathetic activity will increase.

    e. Central venous pressure will increase.

10–12. Which of the following represents a normal compensatory response to chronic endurance exercise training?

    a. an increase in circulating blood volume

    b. an increase in the resting heart rate

    c. an increase in mean arterial pressure

    d. a decrease in resting stroke volume

    e. a decrease in resting blood flow to the kidneys

10–13. Total systemic peripheral vascular resistance of a newborn baby undergoes an abrupt and sustained increase at birth. This is because

    a. Circulating blood volume increases.

    b. The high-resistance lungs inflate.

    c. The low-resistance placental circulation is removed.

    d. Sympathetic neural stimulation is elevated.

    e. Cardiac output rises.

Cardiovascular Function in Pathological Situations

11

OBJECTIVES

The student understands the primary disturbances, compensatory responses, decompensatory processes, and possible therapeutic interventions that pertain to various abnormal cardiovascular situations.

▶ Defines circulatory shock.

▶ Identifies the primary disturbances that can account for cardiogenic, hypovolemic, anaphylactic, septic, and neurogenic shock states.

▶ Lists the compensatory processes that may arise during shock.

▶ Identifies the decompensatory processes that may arise during shock and describes how these lead to irreversible shock states.

▶ Indicates how coronary artery disease may lead to abnormal cardiac function.

▶ Defines the term angina pectoris and describes the mechanisms that promote its development.

▶ Indicates the mechanisms by which various therapeutic interventions may alleviate angina and myocardial ischemia in association with coronary artery disease.

▶ Defines the term heart failure and differentiates between systolic and diastolic dysfunction.

▶ Identifies the short-term and long-term compensatory processes that accompany heart failure.

▶ Describes the advantages and disadvantages of the fluid accumulation that accompanies heart failure.

▶ Defines pulmonary and systemic arterial hypertension.

▶ Identifies the various factors that may contribute to the development of systemic hypertension.

▶ Describes the role of the kidney in establishing and/or maintaining systemic hypertension.

In this last chapter, some of the pathological situations that can interfere with the homeostatic functions of the cardiovascular system are introduced. It is not intended as an in-depth coverage of cardiovascular diseases but rather as an introductory presentation of how the physiological processes described previously are evoked and/or altered during various abnormal cardiovascular states. In each case there is generally a primary disturbance that evokes appropriate compensatory reflex responses. Often, however, pathological situations also lead to inappropriate "decompensatory processes," which tend to accelerate the deterioration of cardiovascular function. Therapeutic interventions may be required and are often designed to limit or reverse these decompensatory processes. Students are again encouraged to review the summary of cardiovascular variables and their determinants in Appendix C because a thorough knowledge of this material will greatly help to understand the physiological consequences of these abnormalities.

CIRCULATORY SHOCK

A state of circulatory shock exists whenever there is a generalized, severe reduction in blood supply to the body tissues and the metabolic needs of the tissues are not met. Even with all cardiovascular compensatory mechanisms activated, arterial pressure is usually (though not always) low in shock.

Primary Disturbances

In general, the shock state is precipitated either by severely depressed myocardial functional ability, by grossly inadequate cardiac filling due to low mean circulatory filling pressure or by profound systemic vasodilation. The first situation is called *cardiogenic shock* and occurs whenever cardiac pumping ability is compromised (eg, severe arrhythmias, abrupt valve malfunction, coronary occlusions, and myocardial infarction). The latter situations can be caused by any of the conditions itemized as follows that decrease central venous volume, ventricular filling or total peripheral resistance:

1. *Hypovolemic shock* accompanies significant hemorrhage (usually greater than 20% of blood volume), severe burns, chronic diarrhea, or prolonged vomiting. These situations can induce shock by depleting body fluids and thus circulating blood volume.

    The occurrence of a *pulmonary embolus* (a clot mobilized from systemic veins lodging in a pulmonary vessel) may evoke a shock state that resembles hypovolemic shock in that left ventricular filling may be compromised. Although small emboli have minor functional consequences, large emboli not only reduce cardiac output but also interfere with adequate gas exchange in the lungs.

2. *Anaphylactic shock* occurs as a result of a severe allergic reaction to an antigen to which the patient has developed a sensitivity (eg, insect bites, antibiotics, and certain foods). This immunological event, also called an "immediate hypersensitivity reaction," is mediated by several substances (such as histamine, prostaglandins, leukotrienes, and bradykinin) that, by multiple mechanisms not well understood, results in substantial peripheral vasodilation with reduction in total peripheral resistance and increases microvascular permeability.

3. *Septic shock* is caused by vasodilator effects of substances released into the circulating blood by infective agents. One of the most common is *endotoxin*, a lipopolysaccharide released from bacteria. This substance induces the formation

of a nitric oxide synthase (called *inducible* nitric oxide synthase to distinguish it from the normally present *constitutive* nitric oxide synthase) in endothelial cells, vascular smooth muscle, and macrophages that then produce large amounts of the potent vasodilator nitric oxide.

4. *Neurogenic shock* is produced by loss of vascular tone due to inhibition of the normal tonic activity of the sympathetic vasoconstrictor nerves and often occurs with deep general anesthesia or in reflex response to deep pain associated with traumatic injuries. The transient vasovagal syncope that may be evoked by strong emotions is a mild form of neurogenic shock.

As shown in the top half of Figure 11–1, the common primary disturbances in all forms of shock are decreased cardiac output and decreased mean arterial pressure. Generally, the reduction in arterial pressure is substantial, and so, therefore, is the influence on the cardiovascular centers from reduced arterial baroreceptor discharge rate. In addition, in the case of hypovolemic, anaphylactic, and septic shock, diminished activity of the cardiopulmonary baroreceptors due to a decrease in central venous pressure and/or volume acts on the medullary cardiovascular centers to stimulate sympathetic output.[1] If arterial pressure falls below approximately 60 mmHg, brain blood flow begins to fall and this elicits the cerebral ischemic response. As indicated in Chapter 9, the cerebral ischemic response causes the most intense of all activation of the sympathetic nerves.

Compensatory Mechanisms

In general, the various forms of shock elicit the compensatory responses in the autonomic nervous system that we would expect from a fall in blood pressure.[2] These are indicated in the bottom half of Figure 11–1. These compensatory responses to shock, however, may be much more intense than those that accompany more ordinary cardiovascular disturbances. Many of the commonly recognized symptoms of shock (eg, pallor, cold clammy skin, rapid heart rate, muscle weakness, and venous constriction) are a result of greatly increased sympathetic nerve activity. When the immediate compensatory processes are inadequate, the individual may also show signs of abnormally low arterial pressure, such as dizziness, confusion, or loss of consciousness.

There are some additional compensatory processes that are initiated during the shock state:

1. Breathing is rapid and may be shallow, which promotes venous return to the heart by action of the respiratory pump.

---

[1] In the case of cardiogenic shock, central venous pressure will increase; and in the case of neurogenic shock, central venous pressure cannot be predicted because both cardiac output and venous return are likely to be depressed. Thus, in these instances, it is not clear how the cardiopulmonary baroreceptors affect autonomic output.

[2] Two primary exceptions to this statement include (1) neurogenic shock, where reflex responses may be absent or lead to further depression of blood pressure, and (2) certain instances of cardiogenic shock associated with inferoposterior myocardial infarctions, which elicit a reflex bradycardia and decrease sympathetic drive (the Bezold–Jarisch reflex).

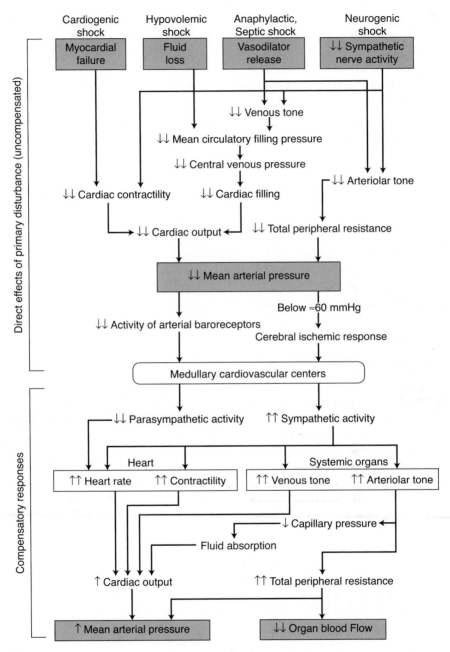

Figure 11–1. Cardiovascular alterations in shock.

2. The release of renin from the kidney as a result of sympathetic stimulation promotes the formation of the hormone, angiotensin II, which is a potent vasoconstrictor and participates in the increase in total peripheral resistance even in mild shock states.

3. The circulating level of vasopressin (also known as, antidiuretic hormone) from the posterior pituitary gland increases and, being a potent vasoconstrictor, contributes to the increase in total peripheral resistance. This hormone is released in response to decreased firing of the cardiopulmonary and arterial baroreceptors.

4. Circulating levels of epinephrine from the adrenal medulla increase in response to sympathetic stimulation and contribute to the vasoconstriction.

5. The increase in arteriolar constriction reduces capillary hydrostatic pressure. Because plasma oncotic pressure has not changed (at least initially), there is a net shift of fluid from the interstitial space into the vascular space.

6. Glycogenolysis in the liver induced by epinephrine and norepinephrine results in a release of glucose and a rise in blood (and interstitial) glucose levels and, more importantly, a rise in extracellular osmolarity by as many as 20 mOsm. This will induce a shift of fluid from the intracellular space into the extracellular (including intravascular) space.

The latter two processes result in a sort of "autotransfusion" that can move as much as a liter of fluid into the vascular space in the first hour after the onset of the shock episode. This fluid shift accounts for the reduction in hematocrit that is commonly observed in hemorrhagic shock.

In addition to the immediate compensatory responses shown in Figure 11–1, fluid retention mechanisms are evoked by hypovolemic states that affect the situation in the long term. The production and release of the antidiuretic hormone (vasopressin) from the posterior pituitary promote water retention by the kidneys. Furthermore, activation of the renin–angiotensin–aldosterone pathway promotes renal sodium retention (via aldosterone) and the thirst sensation and drinking behavior (via angiotensin II). These processes contribute to the replenishment of extracellular fluid volume within a few days of the shock episode.

Decompensatory Processes

Often the strong compensatory responses elicited during shock are capable of preventing drastic reductions in arterial pressure. However, because the compensatory mechanisms involve intense arteriolar vasoconstriction, perfusion of tissues other than the heart and brain may be inadequate despite nearly normal arterial pressure. For example, blood flow through organs such as the liver and kidneys may be reduced nearly to zero by intense sympathetic activation. The possibility of permanent renal or hepatic ischemic damage is a very real concern even in seemingly mild shock situations. Patients who have apparently recovered from a state of shock may die several days later because of renal failure and uremia.

The immediate danger with shock is that it may enter the *progressive stage*, wherein the general cardiovascular situation progressively degenerates, or, worse yet, enter the *irreversible stage*, where no intervention can halt the ultimate collapse of cardiovascular function that results in death.

The mechanisms behind progressive and irreversible shock are not completely understood. However, it is clear from the mechanisms shown in Figure 11–2 that bodily homeostasis can progressively deteriorate with prolonged reductions in organ blood flow. These homeostatic disturbances, in turn, adversely affect various components of the cardiovascular system so that arterial pressure and organ blood flow

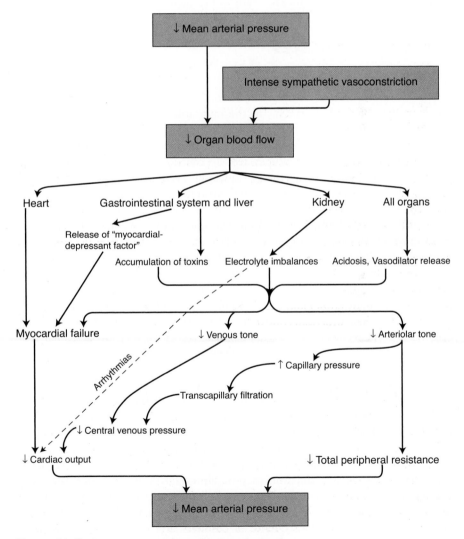

Figure 11–2. Decompensatory mechanisms in shock.

are further reduced. Note that the events shown in Figure 11–2 are *decompensatory mechanisms*. Reduced arterial pressure leads to alterations that further reduce arterial pressure rather than correct it (ie, a *positive feedback process*). These decompensatory mechanisms that are occurring at the tissue level to lower blood pressure are eventually further compounded by a reduction in sympathetic drive and a change from vasoconstriction to vasodilation with a further lowering of blood pressure. The factors that lead to this unexpected reduction in sympathetic drive from the medullary cardiovascular centers are not clearly understood. If the shock state is severe enough and/or has persisted long enough to enter the progressive stage, the self-reinforcing decompensatory mechanisms progressively drive arterial pressure down. Unless corrective measures are taken quickly, death will ultimately result.

CARDIAC DISTURBANCES

Coronary Artery Disease

Whenever coronary blood flow falls below that required to meet the metabolic needs of the heart, the myocardium is said to be *ischemic* and the pumping capability of the heart is impaired. The most common cause of myocardial ischemia is atherosclerotic disease of the large coronary arteries. In atherosclerotic disease, localized lipid deposits called *plaques* develop within the arterial walls. With severe disease, these plaques may become calcified and so large that they physically narrow the lumen of arteries (producing a stenosis) and thus greatly and permanently increase the normally low vascular resistance of these large arteries. This extra resistance adds to the resistance of other coronary vascular segments and tends to reduce coronary flow. If the coronary artery stenosis is not too severe, local metabolic vasodilator mechanisms may reduce arteriolar resistance sufficiently to compensate for the abnormally large arterial resistance. Thus, an individual with coronary artery disease may have perfectly normal coronary blood flow when resting. A coronary artery stenosis of any significance will, however, limit the extent to which coronary flow can increase above its resting value by reducing maximum achievable coronary flow. This occurs because, even with very low arteriolar resistance, the overall vascular resistance of the coronary vascular bed is high if arterial resistance is high.

Coronary artery disease can jeopardize cardiac function in several ways. Ischemic muscle cells are electrically irritable and unstable, and the danger of fibrillation is enhanced. During ischemia, the normal cardiac electrical excitation pathways may be altered and often ectopic pacemaker foci develop. Electrocardiographic manifestations of myocardial ischemia can be observed in individuals with coronary artery disease during exercise stress tests. In addition, there is evidence that platelet aggregation and clotting function may be abnormal in atherosclerotic coronary arteries and the danger of thrombus or emboli formation is enhanced. It appears that certain platelet suppressants or anticoagulants such as aspirin may be beneficial in the treatment of this consequence of coronary artery disease. (Details of the blood-clotting process are included in Appendix D.)

Myocardial ischemia not only impairs the pumping ability of the h produces intense, debilitating chest pain called *angina pectoris*. Anginal p absent in individuals with coronary artery disease when they are resti induced during physical exertion or emotional excitement. Both of these si elicit an increase in sympathetic tone that increases myocardial oxygen consump Myocardial ischemia and chest pain will result if coronary blood flow cannot pace with the increase in myocardial metabolism.

Primary treatment of coronary artery disease (and atherosclerosis, in general should include attempts to lower blood lipids by dietary and pharmacological techniques that prevent (and possibly reverse) further development of the plaques. The interested student should consult medical biochemistry and pharmacology texts for a complete discussion of this very important topic.

Treatment of angina that is a result of coronary artery disease may involve several different pharmacological approaches. First, quick-acting vasodilator drugs such as nitroglycerin may be used to provide primary relief from an anginal attack. These drugs may act directly on coronary vessels to acutely increase coronary blood flow. In addition to increasing myocardial oxygen delivery, nitrates may reduce myocardial oxygen demand by dilating systemic veins which reduces venous return, central venous filling and cardiac preload and by dilating systemic arterioles which reduces arterial resistance, arterial pressure and cardiac afterload. Second, β-adrenergic blocking agents such as propranolol may be used to block the effects of cardiac sympathetic nerves on the heart rate and contractility. These agents limit myocardial oxygen consumption and prevent it from increasing above the level that the compromised coronary blood flow can sustain. Third, calcium channel blockers such as verapamil may be used to dilate coronary and systemic blood vessels. These drugs, which block entry of calcium into the vascular smooth muscle cell, interfere with normal excitation–contraction coupling. They have been found to be useful for treating the angina caused by vasoconstrictive spasms of large coronary arteries (Prinzmetal's angina).

Invasive or surgical interventions are commonly used to eliminate coronary artery stenosis. X-ray techniques combined with radio-opaque dye injections can be used to visualize a balloon-tipped catheter as it is threaded into the coronary artery to the occluded region. Rapid inflation of the balloon squeezes the plaque against the vessel wall and improves the patency of the vessel. This technique, called *coronary angioplasty*, may also be effective in opening occlusions produced by intravascular clots associated with acute myocardial infarction.[3] A small tube-like expandible device called a *stent* is often implanted inside the vessel at the angioplasty site. This rigid implant promotes continued patency of the vessel over a longer period than angioplasty alone. If angioplasty and stent placement are inappropriate or unsuccessful, coronary bypass surgery may be performed. The stenotic coronary artery segments are bypassed by implanting parallel low-resistance pathways formed from either natural (eg, saphenous vein or mammary artery) or artificial vessels.

---

[3] Another method for treatment of *acute* myocardial infarction has been the intravascular injection of thrombolytic substances (eg, streptokinase or tissue plasminogen-activating factors) that dissolve blood clots. This method is most successful when these clot busters are given within a few hours of the infarction.

...lic Dysfunction

...tial) *failure* is said to exist whenever ventricu-
...gh myocardial damage, insufficient coronary
...at directly impairs the mechanical perfor-
...nition, *systolic* heart failure is associated with a
...n of less than 40%. This also implies that the heart is
...*n-normal cardiac function curve*, that is, a reduced cardiac
...n filling pressure. Acute heart failure has already been discussed
... of cardiogenic shock and as part of the decompensatory mechanisms
...g in progressive and irreversible shock. Often, however, sustained cardiac
...allenges" may induce a chronic state of heart failure. Such challenges might
include (1) progressive coronary artery disease, (2) sustained elevation in cardiac
afterload as that which accompanies arterial hypertension or aortic valve stenosis,
or (3) reduced functional muscle mass following myocardial infarction. In some
instances, external causes of cardiac failure cannot be identified and some primary
myocyte abnormality is to blame. This situation is referred to as *primary cardiomy-
opathy*. Regardless of the precipitating cause, most forms of failure are associated
eventually with a reduced myocyte function. Many specific structural, functional,
and biochemical myocyte alterations accompany severe systolic heart failure. Some
of the more well-documented abnormalities include (1) reduced calcium sequestration by the sarcoplasmic reticulum and upregulation of the sarcolemmal Na/Ca
exchanger (leading to low intracellular calcium levels for excitation–contraction
coupling), (2) low affinity of troponin for calcium (leading to reduced cross-bridge
formation and contractile ability), (3) altered substrate metabolism from fatty acid
to glucose oxidation, and (4) impaired respiratory chain activity (leading to impaired
energy production).

The primary disturbance in systolic heart failure (acute or chronic) is depressed
cardiac output and thus lowered arterial pressure. Consequently, all the compensatory responses important in shock (Figure 11–1) are also important in heart failure.
In chronic heart failure, however, the cardiovascular disturbances may not be sufficient to produce a state of shock. Moreover, long-term compensatory mechanisms
are especially important in chronic heart failure.

The circumstances of chronic systolic heart failure are well illustrated by cardiac
output and venous function curves such as those shown in Figure 11–3. The normal
cardiac output and normal venous function curves intersect at point A in Figure
11–3. A cardiac output of 5 L/min at a central venous pressure of less than 2 mmHg
is indicated by the normal operating point (A). With heart failure, the heart operates on a much lower than normal cardiac output curve. Thus, acute heart failure
alone (uncompensated) shifts the cardiovascular operation from the normal point
(A) to a new position, as illustrated by point B in Figure 11–3—that is, cardiac
output falls below normal while central venous pressure rises above normal. The
decreased cardiac output leads to decreased arterial pressure and reflex activation of
the cardiovascular sympathetic nerves. Increased sympathetic nerve activity tends to
(1) raise the cardiac function curve toward normal and (2) increase peripheral

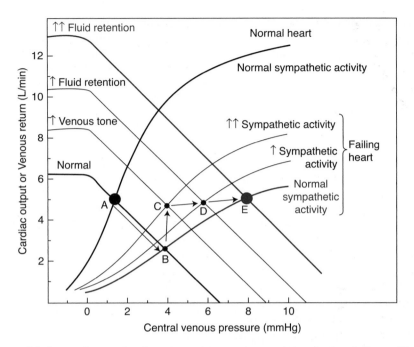

Figure 11–3. Cardiovascular alterations with compensated chronic systolic heart failure.

venous pressure through venous constriction, and thus raises the venous function curve above normal. Cardiovascular operation will shift from point B to point C in Figure 11–3. Thus, the depressed cardiac output is substantially improved by the immediate consequences of increased sympathetic nerve activity. Note, however, that the cardiac output at point C is still below normal. The arterial pressure associated with cardiovascular operation at point C is likely to be near normal, however, because higher than normal total peripheral resistance will accompany higher than normal sympathetic nerve activity.

In the long term, cardiovascular operation cannot remain at point C in Figure 11–3. Operation at point C involves higher than normal sympathetic activity, and this will inevitably cause a gradual increase in blood volume by the mechanisms that are described in Chapter 9. Over several days, there is a progressive rise in the venous function curve as a result of increased blood volume and, consequently, increased mean circulatory filling pressure. Recall that this process involves a sympathetically induced release of renin from the kidney, which activates the renin–angiotensin–aldosterone system that promotes fluid retention. This will progressively shift the cardiovascular operating point from C to D to E as shown in Figure 11–3.

Note that increased fluid retention (C → D → E in Figure 11–3) causes a progressive increase in cardiac output toward normal and simultaneously allows a *reduction in sympathetic nerve activity toward the normal value.* Reduced sympathetic activity is beneficial for several reasons. First, decreased arteriolar constriction permits renal and splanchnic blood flow to return toward more normal values. Second, myocardial oxygen consumption may fall as sympathetic nerve activity falls, even though cardiac output tends to increase. Recall that the increased heart rate and increased cardiac contractility greatly increase myocardial oxygen consumption. Reduced myocardial oxygen consumption is especially beneficial in situations where inadequate coronary blood flow is the cause of the heart failure. In any case, once a normal cardiac output has been achieved, the individual is said to be in a "compensated" state of chronic heart failure.[4]

Unfortunately, the consequences of fluid retention in chronic cardiac failure are not all beneficial. Note that in Figure 11–3 fluid retention (C → D → E) will cause both peripheral and central venous pressures to be much higher than their normal values. Chronically high central venous pressure causes chronically increased end-diastolic volume (cardiac dilation). Up to a point, cardiac performance is improved by increased cardiac filling volume through Starling's law. Excessive cardiac dilation, however, can impair cardiac function because increased total wall tension is required to generate pressure within an enlarged ventricular chamber ($T = P \times r$, Chapter 2). This increases the myocardial oxygen demand.

The high venous pressure associated with fluid retention also adversely affects organ function because high venous pressure produces transcapillary fluid filtration, edema formation, and congestion (hence the commonly used term *congestive heart failure*). Pulmonary edema with dyspnea (shortness of breath)[5] and respiratory crisis often accompanies left-sided heart failure. Common signs of right-sided heart failure include distended neck veins, ankle edema, and fluid accumulation in the abdomen (ascites) with liver congestion and dysfunction.[6]

In the example shown in Figure 11–3, the depression in the cardiac output curve because of heart failure is only moderately severe. Thus, it is possible, through moderate fluid retention, to achieve a normal cardiac output with essentially normal sympathetic activity (point E). The situation at point E is relatively stable because the stimuli for further fluid retention have been removed. If, however, the heart failure is more severe, the cardiac output curve may be so depressed that normal cardiac output cannot be achieved by any amount of fluid retention. In these cases fluid retention is extremely marked, as is the elevation in venous pressure, and the complications of congestion are very serious problems.

---

[4] The extracellular fluid volume remains expanded after reaching the compensated state even though sympathetic activity may have returned to near normal levels. Net fluid loss requires a period of *less than normal* sympathetic activity, which does not occur. For reasons not well understood, the cardiopulmonary baroreceptor reflexes apparently become less responsive to the increased central venous pressure and volume associated with heart failure.

[5] Patients often complain of difficulty breathing especially during the night (paroxysmal nocturnal dyspnea). Being recumbent promotes a fluid shift from the extremities into the central venous pool and lungs, making the patient's pulmonary problems worse. Such patients often sleep more comfortably when propped up.

[6] Plasma volume expansion combines with abnormal liver function to reduce the concentration of plasma proteins by as much as 30%. This reduction in plasma oncotic pressure contributes to the development of interstitial edema of congestive heart failure.

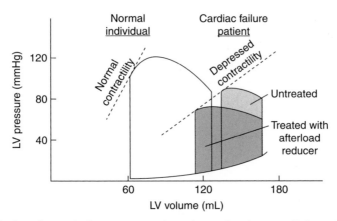

Figure 11–4. Left ventricular pressure–volume loops showing systolic heart failure (loops to the right) characterized by depressed contractility, increased end-diastolic volume, and reduced ejection fraction.

Another way of looking at the effects of left ventricular cardiac failure is given in Figure 11–4. The left ventricular pressure–volume loops describing the events of a cardiac cycle from a failing heart are displaced far to the right of those from normal hearts. The untreated patient described in this figure is in serious trouble with a reduced stroke volume and ejection fraction and high filling pressure. Furthermore, the slope of the line describing the end-systolic pressure–volume relationship is shifted downward and is less steep, indicating the reduced contractility of the cardiac muscle. However, because of this flatter relationship, small reductions in cardiac afterload (ie, arterial blood pressure) will produce substantial increases in stroke volume as indicated in Fig 11–4 and will significantly help this patient.

As might be expected from the previous discussion, the most common symptoms of patients with congestive heart failure are associated with the inability to increase cardiac output (low exercise tolerance and fatigue) and with the compensatory fluid accumulation (tissue congestion, shortness of breath, peripheral swelling). In severe cases, the ability of the cardiac cells to respond to increases in sympathetic stimulation is diminished by a reduction in the effective number (downregulation) of the myocyte β_1-adrenergic receptors. This further reduces the ability of the myocytes to increase their contractility as well as the ability of the heart to increase its beating rate in response to sympathetic stimulation. Thus, low maximal heart rates contribute to the reduced exercise tolerance.

Treatment of the patient with congestive systolic heart failure is a difficult challenge. Treatment of the precipitating condition is of course the ideal approach, but often this cannot be done effectively. The cardiac glycosides (eg, digitalis)[7] have

---

[7] A "tea" made from the leaves of the foxglove plant (*Digitalis purpurea*) was used for centuries as a common folk remedy for the treatment of "dropsy" (congestive heart failure with significant peripheral edema). With the formal recognition of its medicinal benefits in the late-18th century by the English physician Sir William Withering, digitalis became a valuable official pharmacological tool.

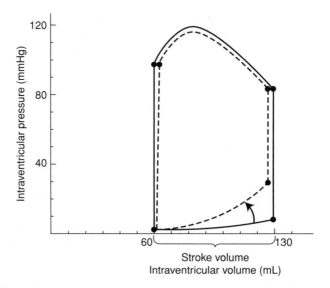

Figure 11–5. Left ventricular pressure–volume loops showing diastolic heart failure (*dashed lines*) characterized by increased diastolic stiffness, increased end-diastolic pressure, and normal ejection fraction.

been used to improve cardiac contractility (ie, to shift the cardiac function curve upward, increasing contractile force of the myocyte at any given starting length).[8] These drugs are unfortunately quite toxic and often have undesirable side effects.

Treatment of the congestive symptoms involves balancing the need for enhanced cardiac filling with the problems of too much fluid. Drugs that promote renal fluid loss (diuretics such as furosemide or thiazides) are extremely helpful as are the angiotensin-converting enzyme (ACE) inhibitors and the angiotensin II receptor blockers (ARBs).[9] A potent diuretic can quickly save a patient from drowning in the pulmonary exudate and reduce diastolic volume of the dilated heart to acceptable levels, but it can also lower blood pressure to dangerous levels.

Chronic Heart Failure—Diastolic Dysfunction

 Although systolic dysfunction is often the primary cause of heart failure, some degree of diastolic dysfunction is also commonly present. As shown in Figure 11–5, diastolic dysfunction implies a stiffened heart during diastole

---

[8] The mechanism of cardiac glycoside action is thought to involve the inhibition of the sodium/potassium adenosine triphosphatase (Na^+/K^+-ATPase) leading to increases in intracellular [Na^+], which is then exchanged for extracellular calcium via the Na^+/Ca^{2+} exchanger. This results in "loading" of the sarcoplasmic reticulum during diastole and increased calcium release for subsequent excitation–contraction coupling.

[9] The ACE inhibitors are very helpful to the congestive heart failure patient for several reasons. By inhibiting the conversion of angiotensin I into its more active form, angiotensin II, peripheral vasoconstriction is reduced (which improves cardiac pumping by afterload reduction) and aldosterone levels are reduced (which promotes diuresis). In addition, ACE inhibitors as well as the ARBs seem to prevent some of the apparently inappropriate myocyte and collagen growth (ie, remodeling) that occurs with cardiac overload and failure.

such that increases in cardiac filling pressure do not produce normal increases in end-diastolic volume. Some individuals (primarily elderly patients with hypertension and cardiac hypertrophy) who have some symptoms of cardiac failure (exertional dyspnea, fluid retention, pulmonary edema, and high end-diastolic pressures) seem to have normal systolic function (ejection fractions >40%), and normal or even reduced ventricular end-diastolic volumes despite increased cardiac filling pressure. Thus, the terms *diastolic heart failure* and *heart failure with preserved systolic function* have been used to describe this situation.

Potential causes of altered diastolic properties in heart failure include (1) decreased cardiac tissue passive compliance due to extracellular remodeling, collagen cross-linking, and other extracellular matrix protein alterations (2) increased myofibrillar passive stiffness due to alterations in the myofibrillar protein titin, (3) delayed myocyte relaxation early in diastole due to slow cytosolic calcium removal processes, (4) inadequate adenosine triphosphate levels required to disconnect the myofilament cross-bridges rapidly, and (5) residual, low-grade cross-bridge cycling during diastole due to calcium leaking from the sarcoplasmic reticulum.

At this point, therapeutic strategies that directly influence diastolic properties are not well developed. Attempts to reduce interstitial fibrosis (with ACE inhibitors and/or angiotensin receptor antagonists) and to reduce diastolic calcium leak from the sarcoplasmic reticulum (with β-adrenergic blockers) have had limited success.

HYPERTENSION

Hypertension is defined as a chronic elevation in arterial blood pressure and can exist in either the pulmonary or the systemic vascular system.

Pulmonary hypertension is much less common than systemic hypertension and less is known about its causes, progression, and treatments. Pulmonary hypertension is designated when mean pulmonary artery pressure is greater than 20 mmHg. It is relatively hard to diagnose until the consequences of the elevated pulmonary arterial pressures (systemic edema, chest pain, fatigue) are fairly well advanced. Right-sided heart failure resulting from chronic pulmonary hypertension is called *cor pulmonale*. Although there is a genetic component to its incidence, it seems to be highly correlated with conditions involving chronic hypoxia (eg, chronic obstructive pulmonary disease, cystic fibrosis, and pneumoconiosis).[10] The increased prevalence of obesity with accompanying obstructive sleep apnea may account for a recent increase in reported incidence of this disease. There is no cure at present and strategies for treatment of systemic hypertension have little or no effect on pulmonary hypertension. However, recent pharmacological approaches using blockers of the receptors for the vasoconstrictor, endothelin, are promising.

---

[10] It is noteworthy that *acute* pulmonary hypertension and pulmonary edema are recognized risks of mountain climbing to extreme altitudes without the aid of supplemental oxygen.

Systemic hypertension is defined as an elevation of mean systemic arterial pressure above 140/90 mmHg. It is an extremely common cardiovascular problem, affecting more than 20% of the adult population of the western world. It has been established beyond doubt that hypertension increases the risk of coronary artery disease, myocardial infarction, heart failure, stroke, and many other serious cardiovascular problems. Moreover, it has been clearly demonstrated that the risk of serious cardiovascular incidents is reduced by proper treatment of hypertension.[11]

In approximately 90% of cases, the primary abnormality that produces high blood pressure is unknown. This condition is sometimes referred to as primary or essential hypertension because the elevated level was thought to be "essential" to drive the blood through the systemic circulation. In the remaining 10% of hypertensive patients, the cause can be traced to a variety of sources, including epinephrine-producing tumors (pheochromocytomas), aldosterone-producing tumors (in primary hyperaldosteronism), certain forms of renal disease (eg, renal artery stenosis, glomerular nephritis, and toxemia of pregnancy), certain neurological disorders (eg, brain tumors that increase intracranial pressure), certain thyroid and parathyroid disorders, aortic coarctation, lead poisoning, drug side effects, abuse of certain drugs, or even unusual dietary habits. The high blood pressure that accompanies such known causes is referred to as secondary hypertension. Most often, however, the true cause of the hypertension remains a mystery, and it is only the symptom of high blood pressure that is treated.

Facts about Systemic Hypertension

In the midst of an enormous amount of information about systemic hypertension, a few universally accepted facts stand out:

1. Genetic factors contribute importantly to the development of hypertension. Familial tendencies for high blood pressure are well documented. In addition, hypertension is generally more common in men than in women and in blacks than in whites.

2. Environmental factors can influence the development of hypertension. High-salt diets and/or certain forms of psychological stress may either aggravate or precipitate hypertension in genetically susceptible individuals.

3. Structural changes in the left side of the heart and arterial vessels occur in response to hypertension. Early alterations include hypertrophy of muscle cells and thickening of the walls of the ventricle and systemic resistance vessels. Late changes associated with deterioration of function include increases in connective tissue and loss of elasticity.

---

[11] Because an increased risk of cardiovascular complications with even mildly elevated blood pressure has been identified, a category designated *prehypertension* has been added to include blood pressures ranging from 120 to 139 mmHg systolic and 80 to 89 mmHg diastolic.

4. The established phase of hypertension is associated with an increase in total peripheral resistance. Cardiac output and/or blood volume may be elevated during the early developmental phase, but these variables are usually normal after the hypertension is established.

5. The increased total peripheral resistance associated with established hypertension may be due to (a) *rarefaction* (decrease in density) of microvessels, (b) the pronounced structural adaptations that occur in the peripheral vascular bed, (c) a continuously increased activity of the vascular smooth muscle cells,[12] (d) an increased sensitivity and reactivity of the vascular smooth muscle cells to external vasoconstrictor stimuli, and/or (e) diminished production and/or effect of endogenous vasodilator substances (eg, nitric oxide).

6. The chronic elevation in blood pressure does not appear to be due to a sustained elevation in sympathetic vasoconstrictor neural discharge nor is it due to a sustained elevation of any blood-borne vasoconstrictive factor. (Both neural and hormonal influences, however, may help initiate primary hypertension.)

7. Blood pressure-regulating reflexes (both the short-term arterial and cardiopulmonary baroreceptor reflexes and the long-term, renal-dependent, pressure-regulating reflexes) become adapted or "reset" to regulate blood pressure at a higher than normal level.

8. Disturbances in renal function contribute importantly to the development and maintenance of primary hypertension. Recall that the urinary output rate is influenced by arterial pressure, and, in the long term, arterial pressure can stabilize only at the level that makes urinary output rate equal to fluid intake rate. As shown by point N in Figure 11–6, this pressure is approximately 100 mmHg in a normal individual.

All forms of hypertension involve an alteration somewhere in the chain of events by which changes in arterial pressure produce changes in urinary output rate (see Figure 9–6) such that the renal function curve is shifted rightward as indicated in Figure 11–6. The important feature to note is that *higher than normal arterial pressure is required to produce a normal urinary output rate in a hypertensive individual.* Although this condition is always present with hypertension, it is not clear whether it could be the common cause of hypertension or simply another one of the many adaptations to it.

Consider that the untreated hypertensive individual in Figure 11–6 would have a very low urinary output rate at the normal mean arterial pressure of 100 mmHg. Recall from Figure 9–5 that whenever the fluid intake rate exceeds the urinary output rate, fluid volume must rise and consequently so will cardiac output and mean arterial pressure. With a normal fluid intake rate, this untreated hypertensive patient will ultimately stabilize at point A (mean arterial pressure 150 mmHg).

---

[12] Continuous activation of vascular smooth muscle might be evoked by autoregulatory responses to increased blood pressure, as discussed in Chapter 6. A *total body autoregulation* could produce an increase in total peripheral resistance so that total systemic flow (ie, cardiac output) would remain nearly normal in the presence of increased mean arterial pressure.

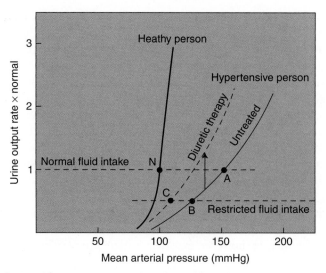

Figure 11–6. Renal function curves in healthy and hypertensive people.

Recall from Chapter 9 that the baroreceptors adapt within days so that they have a normal discharge rate at the *prevailing* average arterial pressure. Thus, once the hypertensive individual has been at point A for a week or more, even the baroreceptor mechanism will begin resisting acute changes from the 150-mmHg pressure level.

A most important fact to realize is that, although either high cardiac output or high total peripheral resistance must always ultimately sustain high blood pressure, neither needs be the primary cause. A shift in the relationship between arterial pressure and urinary output rate, as illustrated in Figure 11–6, however, will always produce hypertension. The possibility that the kidneys actually "set" the blood pressure is supported by evidence accumulating from kidney transplant studies. In these studies, the blood pressure is shown to "follow" the kidney (ie, putting a hypertensive kidney in a normotensive individual produces a hypertensive individual, whereas putting a normotensive kidney in a hypertensive individual produces a normotensive individual).

Therapeutic Strategies for Treatment of Systemic Hypertension

In certain hypertensive individuals, restricting salt intake produces a substantial reduction in blood pressure because of the reduced requirement for water retention to osmotically balance the salt load. In the example in Figure 11–6, this effect is illustrated by a shift from point A to point B. The efficacy of lowering salt intake to lower arterial pressure depends heavily on the slope of the renal function curve in the hypertensive individual. The arterial pressure of a healthy individual, for example, is affected only slightly by changes in salt intake because the normal renal function curve is so steep.

A second common treatment of hypertension is diuretic therapy. Many diuretic drugs are available, but most have the effect of inhibiting renal tubular salt (and therefore fluid) reabsorption. The net effect of diuretic therapy, as shown in Figure 11–6, is that the urinary output rate for a given arterial pressure is increased; that is, diuretic therapy raises the renal function curve. The combined result of restricted fluid intake and diuretic therapy for the hypertensive individual in Figure 11–6 is illustrated by point C.

A third therapeutic intervention is treatment with β-adrenergic blockers that inhibit sympathetic influences on the heart and renal renin release. This approach is most successful in hypertensive patients who have high circulating renin levels.

A fourth antihypertensive strategy is to block the effects of the renin–angiotensin system either with ACE inhibitors blocking the formation of the vasoconstrictor angiotensin II or with angiotensin II receptor blockers. Other pharmacological interventions may include use of α-adrenergic receptor blockers, which prevent the vasoconstrictive effects of catecholamines, and calcium channel blockers, which act directly to decrease vascular smooth muscle tone.

Alterations in life style, including reduction of stress, decreases in caloric intake, limitation of the amount of saturated fats in the diet, and establishment of a regular exercise program, may help reduce blood pressure in certain individuals.

KEY CONCEPTS

 1 Circulatory shock *is defined as a generalized, severe reduction in tissue blood flow so that metabolic needs are not met.*

 2 *The primary disturbances that can lead to shock can be categorized as those that directly interfere with pump function (cardiogenic shock) or those that interfere with ventricular filling (hypovolemia, pulmonary embolus), or those that cause sustained vascular dilation.*

 3 *Shock is usually accompanied by a compensatory increase in sympathetic activity aimed at maintaining arterial pressure via augmented cardiac output and vascular resistance.*

4 *Decompensatory processes precipitated by the shock state are generally caused by inadequate tissue blood flow, loss of local homeostasis, and tissue damage leading to a progressive and irreversible fall in arterial pressure.*

 5 *Coronary artery disease, usually associated with development of atherosclerotic plaques, results in a progressive compromise in coronary blood flow that becomes inadequate to meet the tissue's metabolic needs.*

6 Systolic heart failure *is defined as a reduction of cardiac muscle contractility and results in a depressed cardiac output at all preloads.*

Compensatory fluid retention mechanisms are evoked in heart failure to improve cardiac filling, but when fluid retention is excessive, congestive complications arise (eg, pulmonary edema and abdominal ascites).

Diastolic dysfunction resulting from reduced cardiac compliance often accompanies (and may precipitate) heart failure.

Elevation of pulmonary arterial pressure accompanies acute or chronic conditions of hypoxia.

Chronic elevation of systemic arterial blood is a common and serious condition influenced by multiple genetic and environmental factors.

STUDY QUESTIONS

11–1. Clinical signs of hypovolemic shock often include pale and cold skin, dry mucous membranes, weak but rapid pulse, muscle weakness, and mental disorientation or unconsciousness. What are the physiological conditions that account for these signs?

11–2. Which of the following would be helpful to hemorrhagic shock victims?
   a. Keep them on their feet
   b. Warm them up
   c. Give them fluids to drink
   d. Maintain their blood pressure with catecholamine-type drugs

11–3. What happens to hematocrit?
   a. during hypovolemic shock resulting from prolonged diarrhea
   b. during acute cardiogenic shock
   c. during septic shock
   d. with chronic bleeding

11–4. Left ventricular chamber enlargement with congestive heart failure increases the wall tension required to generate a given systolic pressure. True or false?

11–5. Why are diuretic drugs often helpful in treating patients with congestive heart failure?

11–6. What is the potential danger of vigorous diuretic therapy for the patient with heart failure?

11–7. Why does renal artery stenosis produce hypertension?

11–8. Your 70-year-old, 70-kg patient has an ejection fraction of 70%. Left ventricular end-diastolic volume is 60 mL. Which of the following statements best fits these data?
   a. Stroke volume is approximately 70 mL.
   b. Left ventricular end-systolic volume is approximately 60 mL.
   c. Your patient may be severely hypovolemic.
   d. Your patient may be suffering from chronic systolic heart failure.
   e. These are normal values for someone this age.

11–9.   All the following are compensatory processes that help maintain circulation during states of hypovolemic shock except
   a. hepatic glycogenolysis to increase blood glucose
   b. rapid respiratory effort to promote venous return of blood to the heart
   c. vasoconstrictive contributions from increases in circulating epinephrine
   d. autotransfusion of interstitial fluid into capillary beds
   e. transcapillary filtration of plasma into interstitial space

11–10. Chronic systemic hypertension is usually accompanied by a chronic increase in
   a. cardiac output
   b. the heart rate
   c. arterial pulse pressure
   d. total peripheral resistance
   e. renal urinary output

Answers to Study Questions

CHAPTER 1

1–1. The lungs always receive more blood flow than any other organ because 100% of the cardiac output always passes through the lungs.

1–2. False. Flow through any vascular bed depends on its resistance to flow and the arterial pressure. As long as this pressure is maintained constant (a critical point), alterations in flow through any individual bed will have no influence on flow through other beds in parallel with it.

1–3. A leaky aortic valve will cause a diastolic murmur. Normally, the aortic valve is closed during diastole when there is a large reverse pressure difference between the aorta and left ventricle.

1–4. False. Slowing conduction through the AV node will have no effect on the heart rate but will increase the interval between atrial and ventricular excitation. The heart rate is normally slowed by decreases in the rate of action potential initiation by pacemaker cells in the SA node.

1–5. The blood flow rate through the lungs ($\dot{Q}_L$) must equal the cardiac output (CO) because of the way the cardiovascular system is arranged. $\dot{Q}_L$ is equal to the pressure drop across the lungs (ΔP_L) divided by the resistance to flow through the lungs (R_L).

$$CO = \dot{Q}_L = \frac{\Delta P_L}{R_L} = \frac{20\,\text{mmHg}}{4\,\text{mmHg} \times \text{min/L}} = 5\,\text{L/min}$$

1–6. (a) Since

$$\dot{Q} = \frac{\Delta P}{R}$$

then

$$R = \frac{\Delta P}{\dot{Q}}$$

224

Therefore,

$$R = \frac{100 \, \text{mmHg}}{5 \, \text{mL/min}}$$
$$= 20 \, \text{mmHg} \times \text{min/mL}$$

(b) According to Poiseuille's equation,

$$\dot{Q} = \Delta P \frac{\pi r^4}{8 \, L} \frac{1}{\eta}$$

With other factors constant

$$\dot{Q} \propto r^4$$

Thus doubling the radius with exercise increases flow 16-fold over that at rest. Therefore,

$$\dot{Q} = 16 \times 5 \, \text{mL/min}$$
$$= 80 \, \text{mL/min during exercise}$$

(c) Since

$$R = \frac{\Delta P}{\dot{Q}}$$

we have

$$R = \frac{100 \, \text{mmHg}}{80 \, \text{mL/min}}$$
$$= 1.25 \, \text{mmHg} \times \text{min/mL}$$

1–7. Significant blood loss has a profound negative effect on cardiac pumping because there is not enough blood left to fill the heart properly. This results in decreased cardiac output because of Starling's law of the heart. The consequence of decreased cardiac pumping ability is a lessened pressure difference between arteries and veins. Because of the basic flow equation, less ΔP causes less flow through the systemic organs. Interstitial homeostasis is compromised when there is abnormally low blood flow through capillaries. Improper interstitial conditions impair nerve function and cognitive ability in the brain and cause weakness in skeletal muscles.

1–8. Norepinephrine is the normal sympathetic neurotransmitter substance, so the same cardiovascular effects that normally accompany activation of sympathetic nerves should be predicted. These include increased heart rate, increased forcefulness of cardiac contraction, arteriolar constriction, and venous constriction.

1–9. Arteriolar and venous constriction would be expected because the sympathetic nerve effects on these vessels are normally mediated via α-receptors. There would be no direct effects on the heart expected because the sympathetic effects on the heart are mediated by β-receptors.

1–10. Among other effects, the β-adrenergic receptor blockade tends to reduce the heart rate and the forcefulness of ventricular contraction. Both these results tend to decrease cardiac output. The β-receptor blockade does not directly influence the arteriolar smooth muscle and thus does not directly change the resistance to flow through the systemic vasculature. According to the basic flow equation, less flow through a constant resistance implies a smaller pressure difference exists $(\Delta P = \dot{Q} \times R)$. Because the venous pressure is normally 0 mmHg, and ΔP is arterial minus venous pressure, this translates to a lowered arterial pressure.

1–11. Plasma sodium concentration will be 140 mEq/L because serum is just plasma minus a few clotting proteins. Interstitial sodium ion concentration will also be 140 mEq/L because sodium ions are in diffusional equilibrium across capillary walls. Intracellular sodium ion concentration cannot be predicted because sodium is actively pumped out of all cells.

1–12. Severe dehydration that often accompanies loss of body fluids results in a decrease in the fluid volume of all body components, including the plasma volume. In this situation, because blood cells are not lost, hematocrit will increase.

1–13. e

1–14. a

1–15. e

CHAPTER 2

2–1. a. The potassium equilibrium potential will become less negative because a lower electrical potential is required to balance the decreased tendency for net K^+ diffusion out of the cell. $[E_{eqK+} = (-61.5\,\text{mV})\log([K^+]_i/[K^+]_o)]$

b. Because the resting membrane is most permeable to K^+, the resting membrane potential is always close to the K^+ equilibrium potential. Lowering the absolute value of the K^+ equilibrium potential will undoubtedly also lower the absolute resting membrane potential (ie, depolarize the cells).

c. Two things happen when the resting membrane potential is decreased: (1) the potential is closer to the threshold potential, which should increase excitability, and (2) the fast sodium channels become inactivated, making the cell less excitable. Thus, small increases in $[K^+]_o$ may increase excitability, whereas large increases in $[K^+]_o$ decrease excitability.

2–2. Elevations in extracellular potassium depolarize cardiac muscle cell membranes as can be ascertained from the Nernst equation (see study question 2–1). This depolarization will inactivate sodium and calcium channels, making the cells inexcitable and thus relaxing the heart. This significantly reduces oxygen demands and helps protect the heart tissue against hypoxic injury.

2–3. a. Sodium channel blockers delay the opening of the fast sodium channels in cardiac myocytes. This will slow the rate of depolarization during the action potential (phase 0), which will in turn slow conduction velocity. This results in a prolongation of the PR interval and a widening of the QRS complex.
   b. Calcium channel blockers slow the firing rate of SA nodal cells by blocking the calcium component of the diastolic depolarization. They will reduce the rate of rise of the AV nodal cell action potential (which is largely due to calcium entry into the cells) and slow the rate of conduction through the AV node. In addition, calcium channel blockers will decrease the amount of calcium made available to the contractile machinery during excitation–contraction coupling and thus will decrease the tension-producing capabilities of the cardiac muscle cell.
   c. Potassium channel blockers inhibit the delayed increase in potassium permeability that contributes importantly to the initiation and rate of repolarization of the cardiac myocyte. This prolongs the duration of the plateau phase of the action potential, prolongs the QT interval of the ECG, and prolongs the effective refractory period of the cell.

2–4. False. It is true that increases in sympathetic activity will increase the heart rate (a positive chronotropic effect). However, the electrical refractory period of cardiac cells extends throughout the duration of the cell's contraction. This prevents individual twitches from ever occurring so closely together that they could summate into a tetanic state.

2–5. The correct answers are a and c. Increases in preload increase the amount of shortening by increasing the starting length of the muscle, whereas increases in contractility increase the amount of shortening from a given starting length. Increases in afterload limit the amount of shortening because of an increase tension requirement. (See Figures 2–9 and 2–10.)

2–6. b

2–7. e

2–8. c

CHAPTER 3

3–1. The ventricular systolic pressure is also 24 mmHg because the normal pulmonic valve provides negligible resistance to flow during ejection. The right ventricular diastolic pressure, however, is determined by systemic venous pressure and will be close to 0 mmHg.

3–2. False. Although there may be minor beat-to-beat inequalities, the average stroke volumes of the right and left ventricles must be equal or blood would accumulate in the pulmonic or systemic circulation.

3–3. All of them are correct answers: a, by increasing preload; b, by decreasing afterload; and c and d, by augmenting contractility.

3–4. One cannot tell from the information given because the two alterations would have opposite effects on cardiac output. A complete set of ventricular function curves, as well as quantitative information about the changes in filling pressure and sympathetic tone, would be necessary to answer the question. (See Figure 3–8.)

3–5. True. (See Figure 3–6.)

3–6. b

3–7. a

3–8. b

CHAPTER 4

4–1. $\dot{Q} = \dfrac{\dot{V}_{O_2}}{[O_2]_{SA} - [O_2]_{PA}}$

$\quad = \dfrac{600\,\text{mL/min}}{(200 - 140)\,\text{mL/L}}$

$\quad = 10\,\text{L/min}$

4–2. Ejection fraction is 0.66 or 66%, which is within a normal range.

4–3. The correct answer is c.

4–4. The correct answer is b. According to the standard ECG polarity conventions, the P, R, and T waves will normally all be downward deflections on lead aVR.

4–5. According to the electrocardiographic conventions, the electrical axis is at 45 degrees and falls within the normal range (in the patient's lower left quadrant). The smallest amplitude deflection will occur on the lead to which the electrical axis is most perpendicular. Lead III and lead aVL are both within 15 degrees of being perpendicular to 45 degrees and therefore will have equally small deflections.

4–6. d

4–7. e

4–8. c

CHAPTER 5

5–1. a and b, because filling time is reduced; c, if ventricular rate is rapid; d, for obvious reasons; but not e, because ventricular pacemakers produce a lower heart rate, which is usually associated with a larger stroke volume.

5–2. (a) Aortic stenosis produces a significant pressure difference between the left ventricle and the aorta during systolic ejection.
(b) Mitral stenosis produces a significant pressure difference between the left atrium and the left ventricle during diastole.

5–3. Tricuspid insufficiency. With proper positioning of the patient, pulsations in the neck veins can be observed. Regurgitant flow of blood through a leaky tricuspid valve during systole produces this large abnormal wave.

5–4. Irregular giant *a* waves (called cannon waves) are observed in the jugular veins whenever the atrium contracts against a closed tricuspid valve (ie, during ventricular systole). Because in third-degree heart block the atria and ventricles are beating independently, this situation may occur at irregular intervals.

5–5. e

5–6. b

5–7. d

CHAPTER 6

6–1. The Fick principle states that

$$\dot{G}_m = \dot{Q}([G]_a - [G]_v)$$

Thus,

$$\dot{G}_m = 60\,\text{mL/min} \times \frac{50 - 30\,\text{mg}}{100\,\text{mL}} = 12\,\text{mg/min}$$

6–2. Since

$$\dot{F} = K\,[(P_c - P_i) - (\pi_c - \pi_i)]$$

then

$$\dot{F} = K\,[28 - (-4) - 24 + 0]\,\text{mmHg} = K \times 8\,\text{mmHg}$$

The result is positive, indicating net movement of fluid out of the capillaries.

6–3. All do: a and d, by allowing interstitial protein buildup; b, by raising P_c; and c, for obvious reasons.

6–4. (a) By the parallel resistance equation, the equivalent resistance (R_p) for the parallel pair is $R_p = R_e/2$.
Then by the series resistance equation,

$$R_n = R_e + R_p = 3R_e/2$$

(b) Since more resistance precedes the junction (R_e) than follows it ($R_e/2$), P_j will be closer to P_o than to P_i.

(c) The flow through the network (which equals the flow through the inlet vessel) is

$$\dot{Q}_n = \frac{P_i - P_o}{3R_e/2}$$

The pressure drop across the inlet vessel is equal to its resistance times the flow through it

$$P_i - P_j = R_e \frac{P_i - P_o}{3R_e/2} = 2/3\,(P_i - P_o)$$

6–5. Since

$$\dot{Q} = \frac{\Delta P}{R}$$

then

$$R = \frac{\Delta P}{\dot{Q}}$$

and

$$TPR = \frac{\overline{P}_A - P_{CV}}{CO}$$

Therefore,

$$TPR = \frac{100 - 0\,\text{mmHg}}{6\,\text{L/min}}$$
$$= 16.7\,\text{mmHg} \times \text{min/L}$$

6–6. False. TPR is less than the resistance to flow through any of the organs. Each organ, in effect, provides an additional pathway through which blood may flow; thus, the individual organ resistances must be greater than the total resistance and

$$\frac{1}{\text{TPR}} = \frac{1}{R_1} + \frac{1}{R_2} + \cdots + \frac{1}{R_n}$$

6–7. False. Since

$$\frac{1}{\text{TPR}} = \frac{1}{R_{\text{kidneys}}} + \cdots$$

a decrease in renal resistance must increase 1/TPR and therefore decrease TPR. When the resistance of any single peripheral organ changes, TPR changes in the same direction.

6–8. True. Because arteriolar constriction tends to reduce the hydrostatic pressure in the capillaries, reabsorptive forces will exceed filtration forces and net reabsorption of interstitial fluid into the vascular bed will occur.

6–9. True. $\overline{P}_A = \text{CO} \times \text{TPR}$

6–10. False. Increases in cardiac output are often accompanied by decreases in total peripheral resistance. Depending on the relative magnitude of these changes, mean arterial pressure could rise, fall, or remain constant.

6–11. True. $P_p \simeq SV/C_A$. Acute changes in arterial compliance usually do not occur.

6–12. False. An increase in TPR (with CO constant) will produce approximately equal increases in P_S and P_D and increase $\overline{P}_A$ with little influence on pulse pressure.

6–13. $\overline{P}_A \approx P_D + \frac{1}{3}(P_S - P_D)$
$\approx 70 + \frac{1}{3}(110 - 70) \text{ mmHg}$
$\approx 83 \text{ mmHg}$

6–14. (a) Recall that $SV \simeq P_p \times C_A$. P_p increased by a factor of 1.15 (from 39 to 45 mmHg) during exercise. Because C_A is a relatively fixed parameter in the short term, the increase in P_p must have been produced by an increase in stroke volume of approximately 15%.
(b) Recall that $CO = HR \times SV$. HR increased by a factor of 2 (from 70 to 140 beats per minute) during exercise, and because SV increased by a factor of about 1.15, cardiac output must have increased by approximately 130%. [2.0 (1.15) = 2.3 times the original level.]
(c) Recall that $TPR = \overline{P}_A/CO$. $\overline{P}_A$ increased by a factor of 1.13 (from 93 to 105 mmHg) during exercise, while CO increased about 2.3 times.

Thus, total peripheral resistance must have decreased by approximately 55% ($1.13/2.3 = 0.45$ of the original level).

6–15. d

6–16. c

6–17. a

CHAPTER 7

7–1. The correct answers are a, b, and c.

7–2. False. Autoregulation of blood flow implies that vascular resistance is adjusted to maintain constant flow in spite of changes in arterial pressure.

7–3. All, because they all increase myocardial oxygen consumption. Myocardial blood flow is controlled primarily by local metabolic mechanisms.

7–4. False. Sympathectomy will cause some dilation of skeletal muscle arterioles but not a maximal dilation because skeletal muscle arterioles have a strong inherent basic tone.

7–5. Hyperventilation decreases the blood P_{CO_2} level. This, in turn, causes cerebral arterioles to constrict (recall that cerebral vascular tone is highly sensitive to changes in P_{CO_2}). The increased cerebral vascular resistance causes a decrease in cerebral blood flow, which produces dizziness and disorientation.

7–6. It is likely that the increased metabolic demands evoked by the exercising skeletal muscle cannot be met by an appropriate increase in blood flow to the muscle. This patient may have some sort of arterial disease (atherosclerosis) that provides a high resistance to flow that cannot be overcome by local metabolic vasodilator mechanisms.

7–7. High left ventricular pressures must be developed to eject blood through the stenotic valve (Figure 5–4A). This increases myocardial oxygen consumption, which tends to increase coronary flow. At the same time, however, high intraventricular pressure development enhances the systolic compression of coronary vessels and tends to decrease flow. The local metabolic mechanisms may be adequate to compensate for the increased compressional forces and meet the increased myocardial metabolic needs in a resting individual. However, they may not have enough "reserve" to meet additional needs such as those that accompany exercise. Coronary perfusion pressure may also be decreased if the systemic arterial pressure is lower than normal.

7–8. b

7–9. c

7–10. a

CHAPTER 8

8–1. None of the choices are correct. (The very small change in vascular volume that accompanies a decrease in arteriolar tone is not sufficient to have a significant effect on mean circulatory filling pressure.)

8–2. Central venous pressure always settles at the value that makes cardiac output and venous return equal. Therefore, anything that shifts the cardiac function curve or the venous return curve affects venous pressure (see the list of influences on P_{CV} in Appendix C).

8–3. False. The Frank–Starling law says that, *if other influences on the heart are constant*, cardiac output decreases when central venous pressure decreases (eg, A→B in Figure 8–7). In the intact cardiovascular system, where many things may happen simultaneously, cardiac output and central venous pressure may change in opposite directions (eg, B→C in Figure 8–7).

8–4. None. Venous return must always equal cardiac output in the steady-state situation.

8–5. Because cardiac preload *is* central venous pressure, the physician will try to lower central venous pressure. This requires a left shift of the venous return curve. The two ways that can be done are decreasing circulating volume or decreasing venous tone. The former is often accomplished with diuretic drugs, and the latter can be achieved with certain vasodilator drugs.

8–6. e

8–7. b

8–8. a

CHAPTER 9

9–1. a and b will increase; the rest will decrease.

9–2. Carotid sinus massage causes baroreceptors to fire, which in turn de-creases sympathetic activity and increases parasympathetic activity from the medullary cardiovascular centers. Both act to slow the pacemaker activity and allow a more normal rhythm to be established.

9–3. a, b, and d increase mean arterial pressure; c and e decrease mean arterial pressure.

9–4. (1) The influence of sympathetic nerve activity on arteriolar tone will be blocked. Arteriolar tone will fall and thus so will TPR. An α_1-blockade represents a pressure-lowering disturbance on the effector portion of the cardiovascular system.
(2) The effector portion function curve will shift downward as shown in Appendix E, Figure E–2B. (In this instance the effector function curve

may also become less steep, because increases in TPR no longer aid in the production of increased P_A when sympathetic activity increases.)

(3) A new steady state will be established within the arterial baroreceptor reflex pathway at lower than normal arterial pressure and higher than normal sympathetic nerve activity, as shown in Figure E–2B.

(4) The heart rate and cardiac output will increase because of the increased sympathetic activity. The cardiac function curve will shift upward, but the venous return curve will not, because the α-receptor blockade blocks the effect of increased sympathetic activity on the veins. Consequently, central venous pressure will be lower than normal (see Figure 8–6).

9–5. a and d are disturbances to the effector portion of the arterial baroreceptor control system, which reduce the arterial pressure produced for any given level of sympathetic activity. Thus, as indicated in Appendix E, Figure E–2B, the net results of these disturbances and subsequent adjustments to them will be a new steady state at a lower than normal mean arterial pressure and a higher than normal sympathetic activity.

b and c elicit set-point-increasing inputs to the neural portion of the arterial baroreceptor control system that result in a greater than normal sympathetic output for any given level of input from the arterial baroreceptors. Thus, as indicated in Figure E–3A, in the presence of these disturbances, the system will operate at higher than normal mean arterial pressure and sympathetic activity.

9–6. a and c. These disturbances would tend to directly lower blood pressure, which would then lead to a reflex increase in the heart rate. Disturbances b and d have no direct effect on the heart or vessels. Rather they act on the medullary cardiovascular centers to raise the set point and cause an increase in sympathetic activity. Consequently, one would expect b to cause increases in *both* the heart rate and mean arterial pressure and d to greatly increase mean arterial pressure but decrease the heart rate (Cushing's reflex).

9–7. a

9–8. c

9–9. b

CHAPTER 10

10–1. Because capillaries have such a small radius, the tension in the capillary wall is rather modest despite very high internal pressures according to the law of Laplace ($T = P \times r$).

10–2. Fainting occurs because of decreased cerebral blood flow when mean arterial pressure falls below approximately 60 mmHg. On a hot day, temperature reflexes override pressure reflexes to produce the increased skin blood flow required for thermal regulation. Thus, TPR is lower when standing on a hot day than on a cool one. Consequently, mean arterial pressure falls below 60 mmHg with less lowering of cardiac output on a warm day than on a cool one.

10–3. The cardiovascular response to lying down is just the opposite of that shown in Figure 10–3. Therefore, patients tend to lose rather than retain fluid during extended bed rest and end up with lower than normal blood volumes. Thus, they are less able to cope with an upright posture during the period required for blood volume to reach the value it had when periods of standing were part of the patient's normal routine.

10–4. The pressure produced by the water on the lower part of the body enhances reabsorption of fluid into the capillaries, compresses peripheral veins, reduces the peripheral venous volume, and increases the volume of blood in the central venous pool. This stimulates the cardiopulmonary mechanoreceptors and evokes a diuresis by way of the various neural and hormonal pathways discussed in Chapter 9.

10–5. $R = \bar{P}_A/\dot{Q}$. Skeletal muscle resistance must have decreased considerably during exercise because skeletal muscle flow increased 10-fold (1000%), whereas mean arterial pressure increased much less ($\simeq$11%).

10–6. TPR $= \bar{P}_A/CO$. Total peripheral resistance must have decreased during exercise because cardiac output increased threefold (300%), which is relatively much larger than the 11% increase in mean arterial pressure.

10–7. (1) The heart rate during exercise is well above the intrinsic rate ($\simeq$100 beats per minute). This indicates activation of the cardiac sympathetic nerves because withdrawal of cardiac parasympathetic activity cannot increase the heart rate above the intrinsic rate (Chapter 2).

(2) Increased arterial pulse pressure and ejection fraction at constant central venous pressure indicate increased stroke volume and cardiac contractility and thus increased activity of cardiac sympathetic nerves (Chapter 3).

(3) Decreased renal and splanchnic blood flows in spite of increased mean arterial pressure indicate sympathetic vasoconstriction (Chapter 6).

10–8. (a) SV = CO/HR
SV = 6000/70 = 86 mL/beat at rest
SV = 18,000/160 = 113 mL/beat during exercise
[You may recall that, in the absence of other information, changes in SV can be estimated from changes in arterial pulse pressure, P_p. The information in Figure 10–4 indicates that P_p increased 1.75 times (from 40 mmHg to 70 mmHg) as a result of exercise, whereas SV actually increased only 1.32 times (from 86 mL to 113 mL), as calculated earlier. This discrepancy emphasizes that while SV is a major determinant of P_p, changes in other factors, such as the compliance of arteries (C_A), can influence P_p as well (see Appendix C). Part of the increase in P_p that

accompanies exercise is due to a decrease in effective arterial compliance. The latter is due to (1) an increase in mean arterial pressure with exercise and (2) the nonlinear nature of the arterial volume–pressure relationship (see Figures 6–8 and 6–10).]

(b) Ejection fraction = SV/EDV, or EDV = SV/ejection fraction
    EDV = 86/0.60 = 143 mL at rest
    EDV = 113/0.80 = 141 mL during exercise

[Recall that central venous pressure, P_{CV}, is the cardiac filling pressure or preload and is therefore the primary determinant of EDV. The EDV changed little with exercise because exercise caused little or no change in P_{CV}.]

(c) SV = EDV − ESV, or ESV = EDV − SV
    ESV = 143 − 86 = 57 mL at rest
    ESV = 141 − 113 = 28 mL during exercise

[Recall that the primary determinants of ESV are cardiac afterload (mean arterial pressure) and myocardial contractility (see Appendix C). Cardiac afterload increases during exercise and thus goes in the wrong direction to account for a decrease in ESV. Therefore, an increased myocardial contractility, secondary to increased cardiac sympathetic nerve activity, must be primarily responsible for the decrease in ESV that accompanies exercise.]

(d)

Key features:

1. End-diastolic volume during both rest and exercise is approximately 140 mL.

2. Ventricular ejection (decreasing ventricular volume) begins when intraventricular pressure reaches the diastolic aortic pressure and the aortic valve opens. Figure 10–4 indicates an arterial diastolic pressure of 80 mmHg both at rest and during exercise. Thus, ventricular ejection will begin at an intraventricular pressure of 80 mmHg in both situations.

3 and 4. Peak intraventricular pressure normally equals peak (systolic) arterial pressure. Hence, the systolic arterial pressure values in Figure 10–4 indicate peak intraventricular pressures of 120 and 150 mmHg during rest and exercise, respectively.

5 and 6. As calculated in c earlier, end-systolic volume is 57 mL at rest and decreases to 28 mL during exercise.

10–9. The external negative pressure served to expand the thorax and "pull" air into the lungs through the patient's airways in much the same way that the thoracic muscle and diaphragm expand the thorax in normal breathing. This method of ventilating the lungs did not have the adverse cardiovascular consequences that positive-pressure ventilation has.

10–10. Blood flow through muscles is reduced or stopped by compressive forces on skeletal muscle vessels during an isometric muscle contraction. Thus, during an isometric maneuver, total peripheral resistance (TPR) may be higher than normal rather than much lower than normal as it is during phasic exercises such as running. In the absence of decreased TPR but the presence of strong set-point-raising influences (central command) from the cortex on the medullary cardiovascular centers, mean arterial pressure may be regulated to very high values (see point 2 in Appendix E, Figure E–3A).

10–11. e

10–12. a

10–13. c

CHAPTER 11

11–1. Intense sympathetic activation drastically reduces skin blood flow, promotes transcapillary reabsorption of fluids, increases the heart rate and contractility (but may not restore stroke volume because of low central venous pressure), and reduces skeletal muscle blood flow. Cerebral blood flow falls if the compensatory mechanisms do not prevent mean arterial pressure from falling below 60 mmHg.

11–2. (a) Not helpful because gravity tends to promote peripheral venous blood pooling and cause a further fall in arterial pressure.

(b) Not helpful if carried to an extreme. Cutaneous vasodilation produced by warming adds to the cardiovascular stresses.

(c) Helpful if the victim is conscious and can drink because fluid will be rapidly absorbed from the gut to increase circulating blood volume.

(d) Might be helpful as an initial emergency measure to prevent brain damage due to severely reduced blood pressure, but prolonged treatment will promote the decompensatory mechanisms associated with decreased organ blood flow.

11–3. (a) In hypovolemic shock from diarrhea, the hematocrit will probably increase because, even though the compensatory processes will evoke a
substantial "autotransfusion" by shifting fluid from the intracellular and
interstitial space into the vascular space, this amount of fluid is limited
to a liter or less. Therefore, a substantial loss of fluid (without red blood
cells) will *raise* the hematocrit significantly.

(b) In cardiogenic shock, the hematocrit may decrease because compensatory actions evoked to maintain blood pressure may promote a fluid
shift into the vascular space. However, because central venous pressure
(and perhaps peripheral venous pressures) may also be elevated, capillary hydrostatic pressures (and thus fluid shifts) are difficult to predict.

(c) In septic shock, peripheral vasodilation and peripheral venous pooling
may actually promote filtration of fluid out of the vasculature in some
beds (which would lead to an increased hematocrit), but the low arterial
and central venous pressures may counteract this shift so changes in
hematocrits are difficult to predict in this situation.

(d) Chronic bleeding disorders are usually associated with low hematocrit
and anemia because red blood cell production may not keep pace with
red cell losses, whereas the volume-regulating mechanisms may be able
to maintain a normal blood volume.

11–4. True. The law of Laplace states that, when the radius (r) of a cylinder (or
in this case the irregularly shaped ventricular chamber) increases, the wall
tension (T) for a given internal pressure (P) must also increase: $T = P \times r$.

11–5. Excessive fluid retention can induce decompensatory mechanisms that further compromise an already-weakened heart (eg, inadequate oxygenation
of the blood as it passes through edematous lungs, marked cardiac dilation
and increased myocardial metabolic needs, and liver dysfunction due to
congestion). Diuretic therapy reduces fluid volume and the high venous
pressures that are the cause of these problems.

11–6. If blood volume and central venous pressure are reduced too far with diuretic
therapy, cardiac output may fall to unacceptably low levels through the
Frank–Starling law of the heart.

11–7. Because of the high resistance of the stenosis and the pressure drop across
it, glomerular capillary pressure and therefore glomerular filtration rate are
lower than normal when arterial pressure is normal. Thus, a renal artery
stenosis reduces the urinary output rate caused by a given level of arterial
pressure. The renal function curve is shifted to the right, and hypertension
follows.

11–8. c

11–9. e

11–10. d

Appendix A

Normal Values of Erythrocytes, Leukocytes, and Platelets in Adult Human Blood*

Erythrocytes	4.0–5.5 million/μL of blood
Platelets	130,000–400,000/μL of blood
Leukocytes	4000–10,000/μL of blood

Types of leukocytes	Percent total leukocytes	Primary role
Polymorphonuclear granulocytes		
Neutrophils	50–70	Phagocytosis
Eosinophils	1–4	Allergic hypersensitivity reactions
Basophils	0–0.75	Allergic hypersensitivity reaction
Monocytes	2–8	Phagocytosis and antibody production
Lymphocytes	15–40	Antibody production and cell-mediated immunity

*Normal reference ranges vary somewhat with age, gender, and race. They may also vary from laboratory to laboratory. To confuse the issue further, various unit measurements are used to report blood data, and so caution must be used in interpreting data.

Appendix B

Normal Constituents of Adult Human Plasma

Class	Constituent	Amount/normal concentration range
Electrolytes (inorganic)		
Cations	Sodium (Na^+)	136–145 mEq/L
	Potassium (K^+)	3.5–5.0 mEq/L
	Calcium (Ca^{2+})	4.3–5.2 mEq/L
	Magnesium (Mg^{2+})	1.2–1.8 mEq/L
	Iron (Fe^{3+})	60–160 μg/dL
	Copper (Cu^{2+})	70–155 μg/dL
	Hydrogen (H^+)	35–45 nmol/L (pH = 7.35–7.45)
Anions	Chloride (Cl^-)	98–106 mEq/L
	Bicarbonate ($HCO_3{}^-$)	23–28 mEq/L
	Lactate	0.67–1.8 mEq/L
	Sulfate ($SO_4{}^{2-}$)	0.9–1.1 mEq/L
	Phosphate ($HPO_4{}^{2-}$ mostly)	3.0–4.5 mg/dL
Proteins	Total (7% of plasma weight)	6–8 g/dL
	Albumin	3.4–5.0 g/dL
	Globulins	2.2–4.0 g/dL
	Fibrinogen	0.3 g/dL
Nutrients	Glucose	80–120 mg/dL
	Total amino acids	40 mg/dL
	Cholesterol	150–200 mg/dL
	Phospholipids	150–220 mg/dL
	Triglycerides	35–160 mg/dL
Waste products	Uric acid (from nucleic acids)	2.6–7.2 mg/dL
	Blood urea nitrogen (from protein)	8–25 mg/dL
	Creatinine (from creatine)	0.2–0.9 mg/dL
	Bilirubin (from heme)	0.1–1.2 mg/dL

Appendix C

Key Cardiovascular Variables and Their Normal Determinants

$\overline{P}_A = \text{CO} \times \text{TPR}$

$\text{CO} = \text{SV} \times \text{HR}$

$\text{SV} = \text{EDV} - \text{ESV}$

Ejection fraction $= \text{SV/EDV}$

$$\text{SV} \xleftarrow{\text{ventricular pump}} \begin{cases} (+) \uparrow \text{cardiac preload (via effect on EDV)} \\ (+) \uparrow \text{cardiac contractility (via effect on ESV)} \\ (-) \uparrow \text{cardiac afterload (via effect on ESV)} \end{cases}$$

Cardiac preload $\propto P_{CV}$ ("$\propto$" means "is proportional to")

$$P_{CV} \xleftarrow{\text{central blood volume}} \begin{cases} (+) \uparrow \text{total blood volume} \\ (+) \uparrow \text{peripheral venous tone} \\ (+) \text{skeletal muscle pump} \\ (+) \text{respiratory pump} \\ (-) \text{standing} \\ (-) \uparrow \text{cardiac output} \end{cases}$$

Venous tone $\longleftarrow \{(+) \uparrow \text{sympathetic activity (via NE, } \alpha\text{-receptors)}$

Contractility $\xleftarrow{\text{ventricular cells}} \{(+) \uparrow \text{sympathetic activity (via NE, } \beta\text{-receptors)}$

Cardiac afterload $\propto \overline{P}_A$

$$\text{HR} \xleftarrow{\text{SA node cell firing rate}} \begin{cases} (+) \uparrow \text{sympathetic activity (via NE, } \beta\text{-receptors)} \\ (-) \uparrow \text{parasympathetic activity (via ACh)} \end{cases}$$

$$\text{TPR} \xleftarrow{\text{arteriolar tone}} \begin{cases} (+) \uparrow \text{sympathetic activity (via NE, } \alpha\text{-receptors)} \\ (-) \uparrow \text{local metabolites } (\uparrow \text{local metabolic rate}) \end{cases}$$

$$P_P \propto SV/C_A$$

$$\text{CA} \xleftarrow{\text{large artery elasticity}} \{ (-) \uparrow \text{age}$$

$\overline{P}_A$, mean arterial pressure; CO, cardiac output; TPR, total peripheral resistance; SV, stroke volume; HR, heart rate; ESV, end-systolic volume; EDV, end-diastolic volume; P_{CV}, central venous pressure; NE, norepinephrine; ACh, acetylcholine; P_P, arterial pulse pressure; C_A, arterial compliance; SA, sinoatrial.

Appendix D

Hemostasis

Whenever damage occurs to a blood vessel, a variety of processes are evoked that are aimed at preventing or stopping blood from exiting the vascular space. The three primary processes are summarized in the following list:

I Platelet aggregation and plug formation: occur as a result of the following steps:

    A Vessel injury with endothelial damage and collagen exposure.

    B Platelet adherence to collagen (mediated by the plasma protein, von Willebrand factor).

    C Platelet shape change (from discs to spiny spheres) and degranulation with release of the following:

        1 Adenosine diphosphate, which causes platelet aggregation and "plugs" the hole.

        2 Thromboxane, which causes vasoconstriction and potentiates platelet adhesion and aggregation.

    (*Aspirin and other cyclooxygenase inhibitors are anticoagulants because they prevent the formation of thromboxane.*)

II Local vasoconstriction: mediated largely by thromboxane but also may be induced by local release of other chemical signals that constrict local vessels and reduce blood flow.

III Blood clotting: the formation of a solid gel made up of the protein, fibrin, platelets, and trapped blood cells.

    The critical step in blood clotting is the formation of thrombin from prothrombin, which then catalyzes the conversion of fibrinogen to fibrin. The final clot is stabilized by covalent cross-linkages between fibrin strands catalyzed by factor XIIIa (the formation of which is catalyzed by thrombin).

243

The cascade of reactions that leads from vessel injury to the formation of thrombin is shown in the figure below and is described as follows:

A Vessel injury or tissue damage with blood exposure to subendothelial cells that release thromboplastin ("tissue factor").

B The plasma protein factor VII binds to the tissue factor, which converts it to an activated form, factor VIIa.

C VIIa catalyzes conversion of both factors IX and X to activated forms, IXa and Xa, respectively.

D IXa also helps convert factor X to Xa (Stuart factor).

E Xa converts prothrombin to thrombin.

F Thrombin.

    1 Activates platelets (makes them sticky, induces degranulation, promotes attachment of various factors that participate in clotting).

    2 Converts fibrinogen to fibrin.

    3 Recruits the "intrinsic pathway," which amplifies further formation of factor Xa and facilitates the conversion of prothrombin to thrombin by promoting the following reactions:

        a Conversion of factor XI to its activated form, XIa, which then converts factor IX to IXa, which then attaches to activated platelets and converts factor X to Xa.

        b Conversion of factor VIII (missing in hemophiliacs) to its activated form, VIIIa, which attaches to activated platelets and accelerates conversion of factor X to Xa.

        c Conversion of factor V to its activated form, Va, which attaches to activated platelets and accelerates conversion of prothrombin to thrombin.

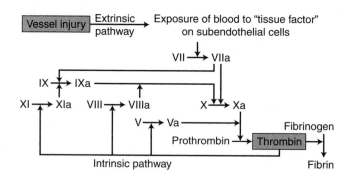

(Several agents clinically used as *anticoagulants* interfere with various steps in this clotting process. *Dicoumarol* and *coumadin* block the activity of vitamin K, which is necessary for synthesis of many of the clotting factors by the liver. *Heparin* activates a plasma protein called *antithrombin III*, which, in turn, inactivates thrombin and several of the other clotting factors. Because calcium is an important clotting cofactor, calcium chelators such as *EDTA, oxalate,* and *citrate* are used to prevent stored blood from clotting. Various *thrombolytic agents* modeled after the endogenous *tissue plasminogen activator (tPA)* are also available that promote dissolution of the fibrin clot after it is formed. These agents promote the formation of plasmin from plasminogen, which enzymatically attacks the clot, turning it into soluble peptides.)

Appendix E

Analysis of the Arterial Baroreflex

For most purposes, the simple "thermostat analogy" provides a sufficient understanding of how the arterial baroreflex operates. However, in certain situations—especially when there are multiple disturbances on the cardiovascular system—a more detailed understanding is helpful. Consequently, the operation of the arterial baroreflex is presented in this appendix with a more formal control system approach.

The complete arterial baroreceptor reflex pathway is a control system made up of two distinct portions as shown in Figure E–1: (1) an *effector portion*, including the heart and peripheral blood vessels, and (2) a *neural portion*, including the arterial baroreceptors, their afferent nerve fibers, the medullary cardiovascular centers, and the efferent sympathetic and parasympathetic fibers. Mean arterial pressure is the *output* of the effector portion and simultaneously the *input* to the neural portion. Similarly, the activity of the sympathetic (and parasympathetic) cardiovascular nerves is the *output* of the neural portion of the arterial baroreceptor control system and, at the same time, the *input* to the effector portion. For convenience, we omit continual reference to parasympathetic nerve activity in the following discussion. Throughout, however, an indicated change in sympathetic nerve activity should usually be taken to imply a reciprocal change in the activity of the cardiac parasympathetic nerves.

A host of reasons why mean arterial pressure *increases* when the heart and peripheral vessels receive *increased* sympathetic nerve activity are discussed in Chapters 2 through 8. All this information is summarized by the curve shown in the lower graph in Figure E–1, which describes the operation of the effector portion of the arterial baroreceptor system alone. In Chapter 9, how *increased* mean arterial pressure acts through the arterial baroreceptors and medullary cardiovascular centers to *decrease* the sympathetic activity has also been discussed. This information is summarized by the curve shown in the upper graph in Figure E–1, which describes the operation of the neural portion of the arterial baroreceptor system *alone*.

When the arterial baroreceptor system is intact and operating as a closed loop, the effector portion and neural portion retain their individual rules of operation as described by their individual function curves in Figure E–1. Yet in the closed loop, the two portions of the system must interact until they come into balance with each other at some operating point with a mutually compatible combination of mean arterial pressure and sympathetic activity. The analysis of the complete system begins by plotting the operating curves for the neural and effector portions of the systems together on the same graph as in Figure E–2A. To accomplish this

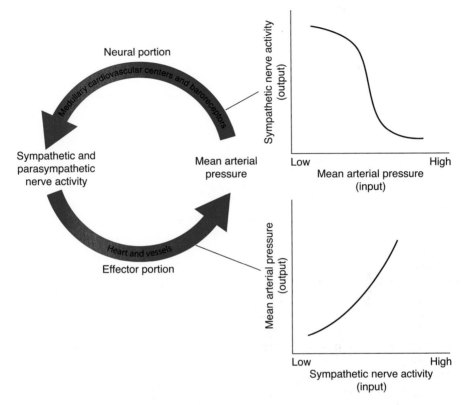

Figure E–1. Neural and effector portions of the arterial baroreceptor control system.

superimposition, the graph for the neural portion (the upper graph in Figure E–1) was flipped to interchange its vertical and horizontal axes. Consequently, the neural curve (but not the effector curve) in Figure E–2A must be read in the unusual sense that its independent variable, arterial pressure, is on the vertical axis and its dependent variable, sympathetic nerve activity, is on the horizontal axis.

Whenever there is any outside disturbance on the cardiovascular system, the operating point of the arterial baroreceptor system shifts. This happens because *all* cardiovascular disturbances cause a shift in one or the other of the two curves in Figure E–2A. For example, Figure E–2B shows how the operating point for the arterial baroreceptor system is shifted by a cardiovascular disturbance that lowers the operating curve of the effector portion. The disturbance in this case could be anything that reduces the arterial pressure produced by the heart and vessels *at each given level of sympathetic activity.* Blood loss, for example, is such a disturbance because it lowers central venous pressure and, through Starling's law, lowers cardiac output and thus mean arterial pressure at any given level of cardiac sympathetic nerve activity. Metabolic vasodilation of arterioles in exercising skeletal muscle is another example of a pressure-lowering disturbance on the effector portion of the

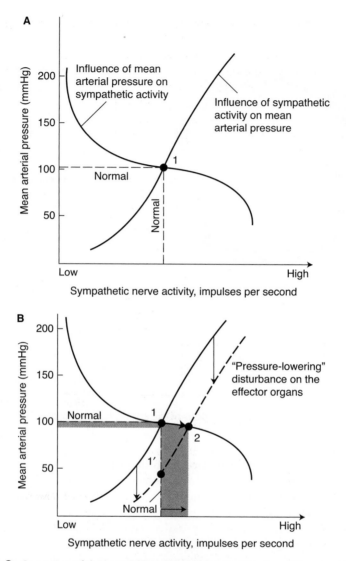

A

Mean arterial pressure (mmHg)

200 — Influence of mean
arterial pressure on
sympathetic activity

Influence of sympathetic
activity on mean
arterial pressure

150 —

100 — · 1

Normal

Normal

50 —

Low   High

Sympathetic nerve activity, impulses per second

B

Mean arterial pressure (mmHg)

200 —

"Pressure-lowering"
disturbance on the
effector organs

150 —

Normal   · 1

100 —

· 2

· 1′

50 —

Normal

Low   High

Sympathetic nerve activity, impulses per second

Figure E–2. Operation of the arterial baroreceptor control system: (**A**) normal balance and (**B**) operating point shift with disturbance on the effector portion.

system because it lowers the total peripheral resistance and thus the arterial pressure that the heart and vessels produce at any given level of sympathetic nerve activity.

As shown by point 2 in Figure E–2B, any pressure-lowering disturbance on the heart or vessels causes a new balance to be reached within the baroreceptor system at a slightly lower than normal mean arterial pressure and a higher than normal sympathetic activity level. Note that the point 1′ in Figure E–2B indicates how far the mean arterial pressure would have fallen as a consequence of the disturbance, had not the sympathetic activity been automatically increased above normal by the arterial baroreceptor system.

As indicated previously in this chapter, many disturbances act on the neural portion of the arterial baroreceptor system rather than directly on the heart or vessels. These disturbances shift the operating point of the cardiovascular system because they alter the operating curve of the neural portion of the system. For example, the influences listed in Figure 9–4 that raise the set point for arterial pressure do so by shifting the operating curve for the neural portion of the arterial baroreceptor system to the right as shown in Figure E–3A because they increase the level of sympathetic

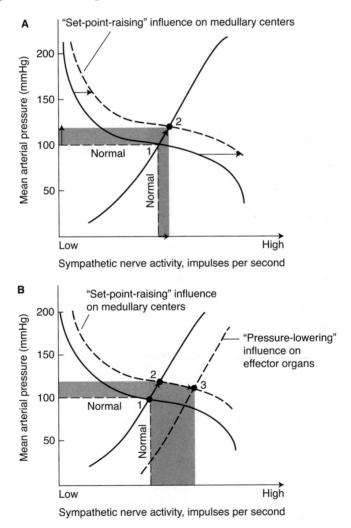

Figure E–3. The effect of neural influences on the arterial baroreceptor control system: (**A**) operating point shift with disturbance on the neural portion and (**B**) operating point shift with disturbances on both neural and effector portions.

output from the medullary cardiovascular centers *at each and every level of arterial pressure* (ie, at each and every level of input from the arterial baroreceptors). For example, a sense of danger will cause the components of the arterial baroreceptor system to come into balance at a higher than normal arterial pressure and a higher than normal sympathetic activity as shown by point 2 in Figure E–3A. Conversely, but not shown in Figure E–3, any of the set-point-lowering influences listed in Figure 9–4 acting on the medullary cardiovascular centers will shift the operating curve for the neural portion of the arterial baroreceptor system to the left, and a new balance will be reached at lower than normal arterial pressure and sympathetic activity.

Many physiological and pathological situations involve simultaneous disturbances on both the neural and effector portions of the arterial baroreceptor system. Figure E–3A illustrates this type of situation. The set-point-increasing disturbance on the neural portion of the system alone causes the equilibrium to shift from point 1 to point 2. Superimposing a pressure-lowering disturbance on the heart or vessels further shifts the equilibrium from point 2 to point 3. Note that, although the response to the pressure-lowering disturbance in Figure E–3B (point 2 to point 3) starts from a higher than normal arterial pressure, it is essentially identical to that which occurs in the absence of a set-point-increasing influence on the cardiovascular center (see Figure E–2B). Thus, the response is an attempt to prevent the arterial pressure from falling below that at point 2. The overall implication is that any of the set-point-increasing influences on the medullary cardiovascular centers listed in Figure 9–4 cause the arterial baroreceptor system to regulate arterial pressure to a higher than normal value. Conversely, the set-point-lowering influences on the medullary cardiovascular centers listed in Figure 9–4 would cause the arterial baroreceptor system to regulate arterial pressure to a lower than normal value.

Several situations that involve a higher than normal sympathetic activity at a time when arterial pressure is itself higher than normal are discussed in Chapters 10 and 11. It should be noted that higher than normal sympathetic activity and higher than normal arterial pressure can exist together only when there is a set-point-raising influence on the *neural* portion of the arterial baroreceptor system.

Index

CCM

Cardiology → invasive
Neph.
IM
Rheum
Heme/onc   Endo   GI

Med/Peds

IM/EM

Anesthesia

ENT

Faves

Kidney
Heart
Liver → lipidology → Diabetes
Blood
Acid/Base Physio
Cardio Physio
Neurophysio → membrane excitability, APs,
                        Autonomics, Neurotransmitters
Pharmacology
Endo

Define

PVR - Peripheral Vascular Resistance

CVP - Central Venous Pressure

RAP - R Atrial Pressure

MCV - mean circulatory Volume

MCP - men Circulatory pressure

3, 8, 7, 6, 11